Some observations o

The laws of diet hold good basically for children and adults alike, but the effects of violating these laws during the years of growth are more profound and decisive for later life.

Nature in her wisdom has given to her product, the whole food, the balance of factors which seems good to her. And therefore we must show respect for this wholeness.

Lean meat as a food is no whole, but a fragment constructed for particular purposes within the whole, put together in a one-sided fashion.

I recognized that the whole marvelous structure of the living substance in the vegetable kingdom serves the purpose of a storehouse of sunlight, or rather of quanta of light from the sun's radiation, and that what nourishes both animal and human life is the sun's energy thus stored in the food.

A diet which is composed solely, or mainly, of foods altered by heat . . . however plentiful and rich in protein, is in any circumstances a defective diet, from which illness will not be far absent.

With regard to the number of meals, let us remember that the Greeks of classical antiquity regarded a man who ate more than twice a day as a barbarian.

the Bircher-Benner
Children's
Diet Book

M. Bircher-Benner, M.D.

Translated by
REGINALD SNELL

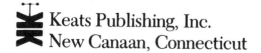
Keats Publishing, Inc.
New Canaan, Connecticut

CHILDREN'S DIET BOOK

Published in 1977 by Keats Publishing, Inc.
By arrangement with the C.W. Daniel Company, Ltd.,
London, England

Library of Congress Catalog Card Number: 76-587-66
Printed in the United States of America
Keats Publishing, Inc.
36 Grove Street, New Canaan, Connecticut

Contents

Foreword

FROM the school's foundation in 1915 the diet here has been arranged on a vegetarian basis. As time went on we became increasingly interested in the outlook and work of the late Dr. Bircher-Benner of Zürich, which, we felt, provided the scientific basis for the way of feeding which the school was practising.

In the spring of 1938 we were able to visit the Lebendige Kraft Sanatorium in Zürich, to see Dr. Bircher-Benner's work at first hand and to discuss matters with him personally. He gave us a copy of his latest book, *Kinderernäbrung*, and as a token of gratitude for all his work for children it was translated by Mr. R. Snell, the Senior German Master at St. Christopher School.

It is our hope that it will be of help to very many who have the responsibility for the care of children.

H. LYN and ELEANOR A. HARRIS,
Co-Principals.

St. Christopher School,
Letchworth.

Preface to the First Edition

THREE conditions determine the constitution, health and later lives of our children: heredity, mental and emotional experience in childhood, and diet. Heredity covers the whole inheritance of mankind and of the chain of generations of ancestors, and the constitutional changes produced by the mode of living, in particular by the diet, of our parents and grandparents. The diet of the mother before and during pregnancy is of great importance. Mental and emotional experience is conditioned both from inside and outside: from inside by the inherited *mneme* and the state of constitutional health, upon both of which things the reaction to the outside world depends; from the outside by the attitude of parents, educators, playfellows and society at large. Whilst the first two conditions, heredity and mental and emotional experience, may be directly and consciously influenced either not at all or only to a trifling extent, the case is very different with the third condition, that of diet. It can be altered at our own discretion for good or ill. Its power is great and goes far beyond all our previous conceptions. "Food is the controlling influence of life and health," says the Japanese investigator, Professor Katase. The statement holds good most particularly for children's diet, during the growing period of life. All parents, therefore, who have the well-being and the future of their children at heart, should be at pains to acquire a sound knowledge of the effects of diet upon the human organism. It is the business of teachers and of educators in general to spread this knowledge and thereby to perform a service of incalculable value to the whole nation.

I wish to thank the Pedagogic Association of Zürich for the suggestion that I should deliver this address, which gave me the opportunity of speaking on June 20th this year to the teachers of that city. This booklet contains the expanded text of my address.

DR. M. BIRCHER-BENNER.

Zürich,

M.O. BIRCHER-BENNER (1867-1939)

AFTER a successful student's career in botany, zoology, anatomy, physics, chemistry and mathematics, Max Bircher took his medical degree at the University of Zürich, and went into general practice in the city. He became interested in the etiology of disease, and was immensely impressed by witnessing the cure of a seemingly hopeless stomach disease, when a patient of his own gained his reluctant consent to try a completely raw vegetable diet, at the suggestion of a quack. He proceeded to try the same treatment on other patients, with excellent results. He began very thorough scientific investigation of the effect on the human body of uncooked vegetables, and finally came to the conclusion that a healthy person should take 50 per cent (and an unhealthy one, 100 per cent) of his food raw. He traced the beginnings of numerous diseases to contemporary "orthodox" eating habits, and—following a medical tradition of long standing, which reaches back through Paracelsus as far as Hippocrates—saw that their only radical cure lay in prevention, by balanced diet. To the teaching and practice of this he devoted the remainder of his long life.

In 1893 he married Elisabeth Benner, and of their seven children three sons took medical degrees and helped to further their father's principles. In 1897 the Bircher-Benners opened a small private clinic, which soon grew into a large and busy sanatorium, visited by patients from all over the world. At first his ideas were ignored or derided in medical circles, but the discovery of the vitamins, and the publication of the findings of modern dietetic research in the early years of the new century, confirmed his teaching beyond all doubt; and at the present time many of his leading ideas—the value of fresh food, the harmfulness of fine milling, the wasteful effects of cooking upon many food substances, the sheer superstition involved in the eating of meat "to give strength," to mention only a few—have become commonplace among educated people. His methods are now part of the regular curricula of several medical schools on the continent, and his books have been translated into eight European languages.

* * *

It may be helpful to add a word about this book, which—although its conclusions are based upon the strictest scientific principles and a wide clinical experience of over forty years—is intended for the laity and especially for mothers, matrons, and teachers. Dr. Bircher-Benner writes a formidable style, and certainly does not make things easy for his readers; I have, however, thought it best not to paraphrase him, but to translate as literally as possible, in view of the extreme importance of what he has to say. Difficult as some of this may sound in English, it will repay patient reading and careful study. His directions for preparing of actual dishes have been made as simple and intelligible as possible by the insertion of the English equivalents to the foods he recommends, so that the housewife or institutional cook who has once mastered the earlier, theoretical sections of the book will find the carrying out of his instructions entirely practicable and straightforward.

Although the author gives no references for his quotations from other nutritional research workers writing in English, I have not re-translated these from the German, but where he cites Drummond, McCann, McCarrison and Hanke I have been at pains to quote the passages directly from their original sources in American publications on nutrition, the British Medical Journal and elsewhere.

I have been fortunate in having the expert advice of someone who is familiar with the technical terms of modern nutritional science as well as the therapeutic side of Dr. Bircher-Benner's work, and with the practical problems of the kitchen—Mrs. Claire Loewenfeld, the distinguished food therapist and pupil of Dr. Bircher-Benner, who is engaged, as this book goes to the printers, in carrying out a diet treatment of a grave children's disease, based upon the Bircher-Benner principles, for one of our great children's hospitals. I owe her my very warm thanks for her generous help.

R. SNELL.

Preface to Second Edition

THE writer of these lines had only just laid down his pen forever when the publishers reported a widespread demand for this introduction to the proper feeding of children. Whereas formerly parents and educators had to be won over to the new ideas, nowadays a vast number want to know how to carry out the diet for themselves. The principles for which Bircher-Benner fought for forty years have become such an assured and integral part of the scientific equipment, not only of our progressive medical men, but of enlightened people in general, that his spirited assaults on the old, and his well chosen arguments for the new methods, cannot fail to move the reader. They require, indeed, to be read over and over again, even by those who are looking, as parents, merely for an introduction to the subject; for the dietetic prescriptions that follow are worthless unless they are properly understood. As editor of the second edition, therefore, I beg the reader to grudge neither time nor trouble to a careful study of the theoretical considerations with which this booklet opens. Only thus will the practical suggestions and examples, which are given in somewhat greater detail in this edition, be appreciated at their true value. It should be emphasized that the process of metabolism in the child depends not only on the food taken, but also—to a greater extent than with adults—upon breathing and movement, and the physical influence of warmth, cold and light; and that therefore none of these factors must be neglected.

In the near future I foresee much joy being given to parents and educators by children brought up on this diet, through their healthy appearance, their increased powers of resistance, and above all their greater educability; I see them growing into strong men and women whose unspoilt sense of taste and strength of character will resist the manias and cravings demanded by a vitiated palate, or a spirit galled by the difficulties of life.

DR. MAX EDWIN BIRCHER.

Zürich

CHILDREN'S
DIET BOOK

The Teachings of Recent Nutritional Research

I

The constitutional health of civilized humanity is subject to a steadily increasing deterioration

HEALTH is a precious gift to mankind. When it is gone we realize the true significance of this simple truth. Perfect health comprises perfect form and structure of the body, perfect functioning of the organs severally and of the body as a whole, maximum immunity from infection and an astonishing power of recuperation after injuries. The profoundest thinker among the physicians of our age, Professor Martin Sihle of Riga, says: "The ideal of health consists in the ability of each individual organ of the body to be equal in a high degree, at any time, to the demands which are made on it, and, as it were, to be answerable for itself."

This ideal of health must be looked for nowadays with Diogenes' lantern. "Through official hygiene," says Sihle, "that is through measures which have been brought to bear upon us from outside, we may have reduced mortality, and considerably lengthened the

1

average duration of life. *But general ill-health, proneness to disease, is on the increase.*"

The diseases of the teeth which are rampant to such a horrifying extent today prove, as Professor Corrado d'Alise of Naples asserts, that "the constitutional condition of civilized man is steadily degenerating." The Japanese nutritional investigator, Professor A. Katase, of Osaka, also declares that "in general the state of man's health at the present time, in comparison with the past, has deteriorated, and this in spite of the great progress in enlightenment and the improvements in medical science and hygienic conditions of life."

All serious investigators of diet have unanimously reached the same conclusions as McCarrison, McCollum, Drummond, McCann, Katase and others, that the chief cause of this constitutional deterioration of our state of health at present is to be found in the defective diet of the civilized nations.

The London bio-chemist Professor J.C. Drummond recently declared in his Lane Lectures at San Francisco: "It cannot be denied that the upheaval of those tragic years [of the European War] drew attention in the most arresting manner to the lamentable condition into which the health of vast numbers of the populations of our civilized communities had fallen. The medical examinations of volunteers and conscripts and the tests of fitness of women for industrial work revealed in England and in other countries a state of affairs which was truly alarming.

"Gradually it was borne home on those who were concerned with the question that defective nutrition was to a large extent responsible for the incapacitating disorders and, for the first time, the extent of malnourishment in the towns of western Europe was widely appreciated. The fundamental truths underlying the aphorism of Brillat-Savarin, 'La destinée des nations dépend de la manière dont elles se nourissent,' became apparent."

We learn from these few utterances of the most prominent investigators the shocking fact, which may be verified in numerous ways, that an increasing sickliness, a growing proneness to disease, is showing itself among civilized mankind. This observation stands in contrast to an opinion which is widespread even in medical circles, that with the decline in infant mortality, the combating of epidemics and the increased expectation of life, a substantial improvement of the general health situation has been achieved.

But many people may find even more surprising the statement which those investigators make concerning the causes of the deterioration in health and constitutional well-being, when they declare defective diet to be to a large extent responsible for it. Fifty years ago it would never have occurred to anybody to attribute such mischievous effects to a national diet that was supposed to have so greatly improved. That such an opinion can exist today is the consequence of a fundamental change in nutritional research, of its transition from purely chemical to biological investigation, whereby results have been obtained which have established our knowledge of how diet is related to health and disease. Forty years ago we doctors knew next to nothing about this relationship.

II

Concerning the relationship of diet to health and disease—The harmonious balance of all food factors

NOT everything which men take as food and drink is nutriment. I am mentioning a well-known fact when I remind my readers that part of it consists of stimulating foods taken for pleasure—among which even cooking salt must be reckoned—and of intoxicants. Furthe·, everyone is aware that the former, if consumed regularly and in any considerable quantity, are prejudicial to health, and that intoxicants are harmful even when they are combined—as in the case of fermented wine—with valuable nutritious matter. There is a reciprocal relation between these non-nutritious foods and diet: the more defective the latter, the stronger the need for stimulants and intoxicants; and the more frequently these are resorted to, the more contrary to instinct does the choice and the combination of diet become. These facts have long been known, but they play their part even in children's diet, although not generally to the same extent as with adults.

The predominant cause of deterioration in health and constitutional well-being referred to, is to be found—and here is what is new—in diet itself.

During the century that saw such progress in the technical industrialization of life, such increasing prosperity, many circumstances were working to alter human diet in certain essential features. One of these circumstances—it must today be regretfully admitted—was the crude dietetic teaching which believed that on the basis of chemical analysis the whole mystery of nutrition had been solved. All this combined to lead civilized nations to a diet on which, as McCollum says, "no race in history has ever yet attempted to live," and which amounts to "an experiment on a scale extending over whole nations," the disastrous effects of which can today be realized.

Certainly this diet is not the only cause of the mischief. We must consider besides such things as the consumption of stimulants and intoxicants, the lack of exposure of the body to the sun, and care of the skin in general, bad air, neglect of breathing, ill-regulated life, late hours of sleep and an excess of emotional excitement—all contributory causes which are linked by invisible threads to the central complex of diet.

The importance attributed, nevertheless, by investigators to diet is a factor in this complex of causes, may be judged from Professor Katase's words: he calls it "an absolutely necessary pre-condition of life and health" which therefore "may be regarded as the controlling influence of life and health"; and he continues: "it is thus the first duty of medical research to investigate accurately the influence of nutrition, that is of nutrients, upon the living organism. Not until the effects of the food consumed by mankind have been properly estimated, will their function inside the human organism be made clear, then a firm basis for preventive measures may be found, and at the same time a signpost for therapeutic treatment set up.

This statement from an investigator of such high standing admits no doubt that the "first duty of medical research" had, a short while ago, not yet been carried out, so that the preventive and therapeutic medical measures which were to be drawn from this source were wanting.

But while even at the end of the last century nutritional research was still enjoying an ill-justified self-complacency, the turn of the century and the early years of the new age brought events both in the sphere of research itself and in connection with the European War, which all at once stirred this research into new life. Effects of diet had been observed which the teaching of the day was totally unable to explain. McCollum says: "A thousand now worked where one had worked before." We may justifiably speak today of a new era in nutritional research.

This era has at last investigated the effects of diet on the living organism, and revealed the connection between diet and health, and diet and disease. Its results, among which may also be reckoned the discovery of the vitamins, were in many points surprising. The inadequacy of the previous teaching became obvious. The effect of diet, it was now realized, is by no means solely decided by the content of the three chief food substances (protein, fat and carbohydrates) and their calorific value. On a diet which contains these factors in full measure, it is still possible to starve. A whole multiplicity of factors, the list of which is not yet exhausted, combines to condition the effect of diet. Diet brings health only *when it combines all the food factors in a natural harmony, in their natural correlations*. Every lasting disturbance of this harmonious balance of factors—an absence, a deficiency or a surplus of one or more of them—causes injury to health.

Science does not yet know all these factors at present, and is not in a position to calculate the natural correlations or to put together arbitrarily any balanced system of diet. But what mankind has managed to achieve has been, and still is, the ruin of the natural balance. Thus we adapted and altered the natural foods with the heat of cooking, baking, roasting and sterilizing. That we were thereby destroying food factors such as certain vitamins, enzymes and so on, and causing not unimportant alterations in their substance and energy value, we did not realize. What severe damage to health may arise through food thus altered we learnt only by its consequences.

Thus artificial feeding of infants with sterilized milk was the cause of the Möller-Barlow disease.* The apes to which McCarrison gave food cooked by steam pressure fell victims within a hundred days to colitis and ulcer of the stomach. Stiner's guinea-pigs, which were similarly fed from the high pressure steamer during investigations at the Swiss Board of Health, fell victims to dental caries, degeneration of the salivary glands, anaemia, scurvy, rheumatoid arthritis, goiter and cancer of the lung. Innumerable disorders of health and illnesses that afflict mankind may be healed by living on uncooked natural food after all the other curative measures have failed.

So, too, we thoughtlessly break up the natural balance of corn grain by the manufacture of finely milled flour and white bread. What this signifies for health cannot be better expressed than in the following words of the London Professor of Bio-Chemistry, Drummond: "Of the many changes which occurred in the nature of food, none had such far-reaching and harmful

*A form of scurvy rickets—Tr.

7

influences on the health of the people as those which affected the character of the bread.

". . . But from the standpoint of public health the modification of the milling process so as to remove the germ was far more injurious in its effect. . . . There are signs, however, that the younger generations of the medical profession are beginning to recognize how great a toll of suffering and ill health the human race has paid for the disastrous industrial movement which has given us the highly milled cereal foods.

"Curiously little effort is being made to produce wholemeal bread or to lead people to adopt it. I am convinced that this will have to be done, and that the sooner the problem is seriously attacked the sooner will be achieved one of the biggest advances in public health that the world has known."

We have further quite one-sidedly overrated the importance of protein, and have in our diet doubled or trebled the amount of it which is suited to man, by laying special emphasis on the provision of foods rich in protein, in particular of lean meat. One cannot rear even lion cubs on the best raw lean meat and bones alone, since they lack at least three vitamins and three mineral substances. For human beings a surplus of protein intake means, as Katase has shown, their subjection to chronic acidosis (i.e. the reaction of the blood is strongly acid).

From certain natural foods, such as sugar beet and sugar cane, we have artificially extracted and "refined" sugar, and now consume it in whatever large quantity we please, without any regard to its natural correlation with other food factors. And acute and detrimental disturbance of the balance of diet, and of our health, is the consequence. According to Katase, "a sugar allowance of only 6 gr. (less than ¼ oz.) a day could be taken without harm by children of five to six years old, weighing about 44 lbs.

Such interference with the harmony of natural foods have we human beings brought about in our unconscious ignorance, but in the pride of our ability and our superior knowledge. The food instinct which every living creature possesses was powerless to protect us, for we had long since turned our attention away from it. Even the soil upon which the food-giving plants grow, we had learnt to weaken through unsuitable treatment, so as to impair in many places the quality of the plants which serve to nourish both ourselves and the animals which provide our milk and meat; and this in its turn interfered with the quality of the milk, the milk products and the meat.

The diet thus wrongly balanced and "purified," combined with the consumption of stimulants and intoxicants, lack of exposure to sunlight, ill-regulated living and the other factors that we have already mentioned, forms a single complex of causes operating in the same mischievous direction, which produces its effects not only in the individual but in the chain of the successive generations. The harm that it does touches by no means only the constitution and the health of the individual, but also the germ-plasm, whereby its effects upon succeeding generations appear earlier and more seriously. From ignorance of this circumstance the inferiority of recent generations is often laid to the account of "heredity," and thus qualifies as an immutable decree of destiny which precludes all attempts at cure. But in reality regeneration is made possible even here, by a removal of the causes—that is, through correction of the errors in the composition, preparation and cooking of food.

Every population today presents a mixture of individuals with varying germ-plasm values, which accounts for the fact that with a similar manner of living some remain apparently healthy while others sooner or later fall victims to disease.

III

The defects of nutrition in childhood, and their symptoms

It has already become clear that the new era of nutritional research provides us with directions for proper child nutrition entirely different from those we previously possessed. It is also sufficiently obvious that *diet influences the period of growth with peculiar intensity*. McCarrison gives expression to the consequent change in our outlook in the British Medical Journal in the following words:

"The truth is slowly being made plain that man is composed of what he eats; that defects in the architecture of the human edifice are largely due to defects in the quality of the food, especially during the growing period of life. These defects are often at the root of disease processes which manifest themselves clinically in later life, but they can be prevented, or when established they can (if not too far advanced or complicated by superimposed infection) be rectified, by correcting defects in the composition and balance of the dietary."

According to this declaration of McCarrison, then, defects in the structure of the human body—meaning for the purpose we are considering the child's body—may be the means of drawing our attention to the qualitative defects of diet. We may even expect and recognize certain functional disorders to be the cause of subsequent illnesses. Since I am probably right in supposing that such symptoms of defective diet will also be of interest to educators, I shall therefore not omit to indicate, at any rate, the most significant of them. Outstanding among the defects of structure are, in the first place, the consequence of rickets, by which almost without exception every child in the mid-European countries, if we take into account even the slightest degrees of the disease, is attacked. Out of our complex of causes, the lack of vitamin D and a wrong proportion of phosphorus and calcium in the diet are primarily responsible here. The problem of vitamin D is of particular interest for the understanding of the nutritional process. This hitherto unknown food factor D is composed of a fat substance, ergosterol, and ultra-violet light. The light content activates the ergosterol, and gives the whole structure the capacity of rendering feasible the hardening of the growing bones through a storing up of lime. In the diet, ergosterol is taken as the preliminary stage of the vitamin D. It is stored up in the skin as in a depository. The same thing occurs also with other substances in an inactive state. The light which penetrates the skin activates these substances, whereby vitamin D is produced from the ergosterol, and now exercises its influence upon growth.

The existence of vitamin D teaches us also that the sun's rays may be ranked as an important vital factor in the nutrition of mankind, and particularly of the child.

That vitamin D can occur also in an active state in food, is well known. It exists in unrefined cod liver oil, and in a lesser degree in yolk of egg also. We shall, however, do well to see that children are given vitamin D not only from these sources, but above all from the most natural and certain source, the exposure of their bodies to the sunlight.

This subject of the cause of rickets is, however, not exhausted by considerations of children's diet and exposure to the sun: we must further consider the diet of the parents and in particular that of the mothers during pregnancy. This accounts for the fact that even infants at the breast may sicken with rickets.

The consequences of this nutritional disease are manifested primarily in the bony structure of the skeleton. Its formation shows warping, crookedness and deformities; added to these are knock knees and bandy legs, curvature of the spine, flatness of the chest, asymmetrical skull, abnormal placing of the teeth with faulty clenching and diminished power of mastication, and a narrow pelvis which makes child-bearing difficult.

Secondary consequences of a metabolism whose balance has been upset by rickets make themselves felt in the general state of health and of the nervous system. One notices increases susceptibility to fatigue, often a certain idleness and heightened reflex-excitability of a nervous character. In the psychological sphere, considerable abnormalities of bodily structure become the nucleus for feelings of inferiority.

During the years of intensive growth, from the fifth to the seventh and from the twelfth to the sixteenth years, we often find relapses into rickets, the so-called "late rickets" whose manifestations occur just during the school age.

Further serious defects of bodily structure arise, as the researches of Katase show, through that disharmony in the composition of diet which is engendered by a superfluity of the chief food substances—protein matter, fats or carbohydrates (e.g. sugar). The excessive provision of foods rich in protein—of meat, eggs or cheese—of too much fat, of carbohydrates, especially in the form of sugar, in the long run damages the constitution of the growing human being through a dislocation of the acid-alkaline balance in the direction of too much acidity. Under the influence of this acidosis there arise, as Katase tells us: (i) through increased growth in length of the bones the long, thin, narrow-chested type of man, the so-called asthenic constitution; (ii) weak muscular system; (iii) pigeon chest; (iv) "pear-shaped" heart; (v) the undeveloped or infantile uterus, and (vi) a susceptibility to juvenile diseases.

In this sense those children who get too many sweets between meals are exposed to particular risks.

The findings of Katase help to explain one puzzling phenomenon of our age: the increase in our height. "Man is becoming taller," announce the anthropologists. Is this a gain or a loss? Since the diet of the nations in general has altered for the worse during the last century, this increase in height must be regarded as a sign of constitutional deterioration. Hand in hand with this over-stimulated growth in height an abnormal precocity also makes its appearance in our children.

A third group of injurious effects produced by wrongly balanced diet shows itself in the regulators of growth and of bodily appearance, in the endocrine glands (pituitary, thyroid, suprarenal, reproductive and so on). That herein not only important vital functions are disturbed, but the whole bodily structure suffers as a consequence, one may see from the goitrous degeneration of the thyroid gland. It must often have struck us, how frequently today diagnosis centers on "endocrine glandular disorder." That shows how widely spread these injuries are. To some extent they make themselves felt even in childhood as disturbers of health and vitality, and to some extent they are planted during these years as the roots of more serious later complaints. The great causal significance of diet for these injuries is still too little recognized and too little considered. This is not the place to go into details. The researchers of McCarrison have shown evidence that it is just these glands which are harmed by defective diet. That lack of iodine in diet plays a part in the formation of goiter is a fact known to every Swiss. But lack of iodine alone is not sufficient to explain the whole phenomenon. Stiner's guinea-pigs got goiter when they received their accustomed raw foods cooked in a high-pressure steamer. The results of the official enquiry into goiter during the recruiting campaign of 1924-5 are instructive, as showing that the difference of dietetic habits between the Latin and the Germanic populations in Switzerland also produced a difference in the frequency of goiter, in favour of the Germans. On the other hand the splendid success of iodine-salt prophylaxis in the Canton of Appenzell is worthy of the closest attention.

In the course of forty years' observation of a considerable number of diseases of the endocrine glands I have invariably been able to establish the fact that a fundamentally corrected food therapy obtained better results than treatment with hormone preparations, which points to the causal significance of a defective diet.

One of the most frequent and certain signs of injury caused by wrongly balanced diet is caries, or dental decay. Between 95 and 98 per cent of German-Swiss children of school age, and about 85 per cent of Latin-Swiss children, already show incipient caries. At a later age this is associated with shrinkage of the gums,* atrophy or absorption of the sockets of the teeth, and loosening of the teeth in the form of pyorrhea, which similarly shows a steadily increasing diffusion in Switzerland.

One hardly dares to proffer the opinion that the struggle against dental caries with tooth-brush, antiseptic mouth washes and tooth paste remains unsuccessful, because, being based on the incorrect theory of Miller, it does not touch the root of the trouble—applies the lever, in fact, in the wrong place. The cause of dental caries does not lie in defective cleaning of the teeth: it operates from within, through the blood which flows along the fine blood channels of the pulp of the tooth, and so affects the whole tooth; and this cause is, in its paramount essentials, simply the inharmonious composition of the diet. Exhaustive researches conducted by many distinguished writers have at last furnished a complete explanation of this question—I need only mention Mellanby, Guido Fischer, Weston A. Price, McCollum, Milton T. Hanke, Bunting, Johan Brun of Oslo, Stiner, and Katase. Boitel of Vevey and Montigel of Chur report oases of sound children's teeth in Swiss orphanages, where there is natural, simple diet without sweets and snacks between meals. Hanke is the spokesman of a group of dentists who for three years carried out experiments upon 341 children of the child colony of Mooseheart in America, in which the control of caries through corrected diet, with the addition of a pint of fresh orange juice per day throughout a whole year, was crowned with success, Katase says, summing up:

*Arising from inflammation of the gums (gingivitis).—TR.

"Dental caries arises not from attacks of acid from outside, but from the attacks of blood acidity from within. It depends not upon the cleaning of the teeth but upon the excess of protein intake, of fat and carbohydrates—that is of acidosis-producing food substances."

We have then, without any doubt, gone about the struggle against dental decay along the wrong lines, and we are still doing so. In spite of the alarming condition of teeth in Switzerland, our children still find no effective preventive support against the disease which is so pregnant with consequences for their later life. Dentists, of course, know all about the matter. But their influence upon the diet of sufferers from dental disease is paralysed through the circumstance that the question of diet is the affair of the doctor, not of the dentist. On the other hand the doctors resign teeth to the care of the dentist, and have no love, as things are at present, for the unpopular attack upon the dietetic sins of the nation—indeed, they often join in deriding it.

One might reassure oneself with the reflection that it is only the teeth which are at stake, and they after all can be artificially replaced; the injurious effects of defective diet touch, however, the whole organism at the same time as the teeth, and in particular certain organs and tissues of it; and the festering roots of stopped teeth become sources of infection and causes of fresh disease. *Disease of the tooth is a disease of the whole body.* "The organic-constitutional condition of the teeth is," as Professor Corrado d'Alise says, "a reliable indication of the condition of the remaining organs and tissues of our body, and will always be so."

A glance at the teeth give us, as we see, our first significant bearings, as to the state of the general constitutional health and the quality of diet of a child, indeed of a whole nation.

In fact, the nutritional damage which becomes visible in the teeth lays hold also to other parts of the body, where it becomes recognizable in functional disorders. The diminished acuteness of vision, the short-sightedness which so often supervenes during the periods of intensive growth, is not, as many people assert, a consequence of heredity, but of wrong diet in the preceding generations. The same holds good for many complaints of the ear. Such consequences of the deficiency of vitamins—so-called hypovitaminosis—always accompanied by further disharmonies in the diet, occur much more frequently among children than is generally known. They manifest themselves in digestive troubles, loss of appetite or voracity, constipation or diarrhea, in sallowness, corpulence or excessive thinness.

Skin troubles such as eczema, psoriasis, urticaria and facial acne are almost without exception the results of wrong diet, for they yield only to a fundamental correction of the dietetic errors.

Of quite especial importance are the nutritional injuries in the sphere of the organs of circulation, in particular the capillary vessels which, with a total length of fifteen hundred miles, and an inside surface of nearly a hundred square yards, interlace the body as a canal system for receiving food and disposing of waste matter. From this capillary net, permeating its walls, the nutritional stream flows out of the blood to the separate organ cells. The composition of the blood depends upon the diet and the collaboration of all the bodily organs. On the blood depend the development and the condition of the capillary vessels and their walls, and these determine the goodness, the capacity and the speed of flow of the nutritional stream on which ultimately health and life depend.

A magnification of 60 with a microscope enables a doctor to see this capillary net at many points of the skin, especially in the folds of the nails and in the lips, and to determine its condition and the flow of blood in its interior. The pictures thus obtained can even be photographically reproduced. Thus a new method of research has developed during the last twenty years: microscopic histology of the capillaries. What has it taught us?

There are two sorts of injury caused to the capillary net and the nutritional stream by wrongly balanced diet. The first affects the development of the capillary net. A new-born child possesses a network of fine blood vessels, but as yet no capillary loops. Not until the second to the fourth year of life do the hairpin-shaped capillary loops grow out of this primitive net. This development is retarded by the same injurious causes which give rise to goiter, cretinism and mental deficiency as their most serious consequences. Slighter degrees of retardation are expressed in the immaturity of young people even as late as the school-leaving age, and associated with this immaturity there is usually found a diminished capacity in physical and intellectual respects.

This arrested development has for Switzerland, the land of goiter, an unusually great importance. Jaensch and Gunderman have carried out mass investigations among school children in Germany and Switzerland, which have turned out by no means in the latter country's favour. Specially selected secondary school-boys of school-leaving age, strong and of sound heredity, taken from all parts of Germany, show 0 per cent cases of retardation; 1,757 pupils from grammar schools in Germany show 2.9 per cent; elementary schools in

Berlin show 4.85 per cent; a "special school" for defectives shows 17.43 per cent; while in Switzerland the findings are: secondary schools 10.11 per cent; elementary schools 17.92 per cent; in the country population 16.15 per cent cases of retarded development of the capillary vessels! These sensational figures should serve to arouse us at last from our slumbers.

The second sort of injury affects the developed capillary loops. Under the influence of blood that has been abnormally changed through defective diet the hairpin-shaped loops have their shape distorted. They become distended bags and show corkscrew-like twists, contractions or even shrivelling. Professor Gänsslen of Tübingen obtained similar changes in two healthy students by giving them excessive meat diet over a space of only ten days. In such capillaries the bloodstream becomes congested and the flow is retarded, so that the nutritional stream to the organ cells deteriorates. And so the same injury affects all the organs, especially certain individual ones such as the pulp of the tooth, and ultimately its repercussions reach the heart, the arteries and the veins. Thus even in childhood cases arise of circulation troubles, cyanosis,* paleness, abnormal redness of colour, and organic heart disease. In 1912 an official enquiry among children of North American towns established the existence of organic heart disease among 400,000 children. I fancy the gymnastic instructors in our own schools could also furnish a contribution to this chapter.

A further far-reaching consequence of defective diet is the weakening of natural immunity against infections which manifest themselves in a susceptibility to varieties of the "common cold"—catarrh or tonsillitis—and very frequently in tuberculosis. Research

*Blue jaundice.—Tr.

has brought evidence that a complete natural immunity can be achieved only by means of proper diet.

That all these nutritional injuries unfailingly make themselves felt also in the capacities and in the character of the child may be illustrated by the following words of the American McCann. He says: "But the badly nourished child often shows abnormal qualities which clever people call 'evil.'

"Many a little heart pumping impoverished blood to hungry tissues, feeding starved nerves with an unhealthy stream, nourishing a tired little body and a wearied little brain with debased foods goes for correction to the Children's Court, or is 'punished' for the pranks over which it has no control.

"You have seen 'bad' children, 'cranky' children, 'peevish' children, 'cruel' children, 'reckless' children, 'nervous' children and 'delinquent' children. Many of them, after a diet of six months on the food God intended they should eat, can preach sermons to their elders.

"The world disregards the most beautiful of Nature's laws in its consumption of degraded, debased, denatured foods, and then murmurs against God, blaming Him for the prevalence of disease upon the earth."

The sketch of nutritional injuries during childhood which I have so far been tracing is admittedly not a complete one, but it may nevertheless serve to demonstrate the great importance of the question of diet for the child, and for the nation as a whole, a question which even today unfortunately receives too little attention. I can now proceed to a description of the right, healthy diet for the child, leaving out the question of infants' feeding, since their natural and sole proper food is the milk from the breasts of a properly nourished, healthy mother.

IV

The proper diet for children—Indications bearing on the natural correlation of food factors and the balanced combination of human diet

THE laws of diet hold good basically for children and adults alike, but the effects of violating these laws during the years of growth are more profound and decisive for later life.

Therefore what is required before everything else for childhood, and in particular for the growing period, is that the diet shall be properly balanced. That is to say, it must consist of all food factors—the many that are already known and those that are still unknown—in their natural correlation, in harmonious accord.

We know today many nutrients—the primary food substances, the mineral substances, the vitamins and so on—but we do not yet know them all. We have only insufficient means of measuring the relative quantity of each individual constituent necessary to satisfy the human body. Besides, one factor separated from the whole and "refined" is, in its condition and effectiveness, very different from that factor in natural association with the whole food. This circumstance precludes any form of arbitrary, artificial composition of human diet.

Nature in her wisdom has given to her product, the whole food, the balance of food factors which seems good to her. And therefore we must show respect for this wholeness. Researches into the nature of life have further taught us that the creator, ordainer, protector and ruler of life has appointed to every living creature—plant, beast or human being—a definite choice from the whole range of existing foods. In this choice, to which its nutritional instinct is the guide, the living creature finds the balance of food factors that will satisfy its needs. In mammals, among which mankind is to be ranked, there exists a correlation between the structure of the digestive organs, and in particular of the teeth, and the range of foods which is allotted to them, so that from this structure the types of food which are suited to each several species can be determined. Comparative anatomists have therefore divided the mammals on the basis of the construction of their teeth into the following food range groups: (i) frugivorous, or fruit-eating; (ii) herbivorous, or leaf-eating; (iii) carnivorous, or flesh-eating; and (iv) omnivorous, or eating everything, the chief constituent of the diet in question being taken in each case as determining the general designation. Frugivorous creatures feed also, for example, on leaves, buds and roots, and carnivorous creatures on vegetable diet, which they prefer to look for in the stomachs of the beasts they prey on. No carnivore feeds predominantly on lean meat; its food is firstly the blood, then the intestines, then the layers of fat, and only lastly the bones and the lean flesh.

We have then two indications for finding a harmoniously composed human diet from among the whole range of existing foods: (i) the anatomical build, the structure of the human teeth, (ii) respect for the whole food, which warns us against all kinds of manufacture and preparation of the foods assigned to us, whereby the natural correlations of the food factors could be disturbed.

The first indication will be contradicted in all those camps where people still cling to the opinion that meat eating is good and necessary for mankind, and believe that a meatless diet is not satisfying. Although this point of view and this belief are supported neither by science nor by experience, they are none the less passionately maintained. It is this attitude which hampers the recovery of civilized humanity and creates manifold confusion. But when we consider how "all too human" man's nature is, it is an understandable attitude. Meat is not only a food (albeit a defective one), but also a strong stimulant, which is even capable of exciting in the body conditions similar to a kind of intoxication; therefore man's attitude towards it resembles his attitude towards alcoholic drinks.

Sine ira et studio, that is quite dispassionately, this question has been decided by Cuvier, and more recently confirmed by Dr. Richard Lehne in a careful and exhaustive comparative-anatomical study. Lehne sums up his conclusions in the following words: "Quite apart from the physiological findings of nutritional science, which perpetually alter and are always in an unsettled form, comparative anatomy proves—and is supported by the millions-of-years-old documents of paleozoology—that human teeth in their ideal form have a purely frugivorous character."

We have therefore to establish the fact that Nature has assigned to mankind the whole range of the vegetable kingdom for food, and that man finds inside this range of correlations all the various food factors which suit him—in other words, harmonious balance in the composition of his diet.

The second indication we owe entirely to the findings of modern nutritional research. They require us to respect the wholeness of food. This "whole" means every food in the complete state in which it leaves God's workshop, whether as fruit, as green leaf, as root, as grain, as seed, or whatever it may be.

In the range of animal foods only the entire animal—as it actually existed in its life—would form a "whole," Young lions in captivity can be brought up only on living small animals. The Eskimos, too, feed on all portions of the animal—blood, entrails, skin, fat and muscle—and on numerous berries, roots and herbs besides. The Eskimo is withal indolent and lethargic, in consequence of poisoning of the blood through putrefaction in the bowel; he is stirred to action only by the impulse of hunger. Lean meat as a food is no whole, but a fragment constructed for particular purposes within the whole, put together in a one-sided fashion.

It must not be understood by this that every individual plant organism contains all the food factors in their right correlation for mankind. This full food value is attained only through a combination of the total diet from a number of different vegetable foods, wherein the green leaves (e.g. vegetable or salads) are distinguished by their capacity of supplementing the seeds (grain, beans, peas, nuts and so on). For the suitable combination of a complete diet we have the experience of countless ages at our disposal.

Out of respect for the whole food, and—what is of ultimate importance—in order to achieve in our diet a harmonious accord of the different factors, we need to fulfil the following requirements: (i) Vegetable organisms which can be eaten fresh and raw should preferably be so eaten. These include all kinds of fruit, berries, many roots (such as carrots, radishes and so on), leaf vegetables prepared as salads or hors d'oeuvres, vegetable fruits (e.g. tomatoes and cucumbers), nuts and almonds. Careful cleaning of all these is necessary.

(ii) As heat weakens or destroys nutrients according to its intensity and duration, cooked, baked or roasted foods have lost more or less of their wholeness. This applies in a high degree to sterilized preserves, which should be used only in times of need. Mineral substances and other food values escape from the vegetables into the water in which they are boiled, and are lost, as they are in scalding (when the water is poured off). We should therefore curtail the length of boiling, moderate the degree of heat, keep the water used for boiling, and employ cooked food only as an accompaniment to abundant raw food.

(iii) Our diet ought to contain the whole grain with its germ and inner husk. Therefore children should on no account be given white bread, but wholemeal bread. Further, all white flour foods should be allowed them only in strictly limited amounts.

(iv) The supply of sugar should be confined, if possible, exclusively to the natural association of the sugar-containing foods—fruits, honey, root vegetables and so on. The manufacture of refined sugar tears this away from its association (and correlation) with other food factors. Any considerable consumption of refined sugar means a disturbance of the nutritional balance which may lead to serious consequences. The giving to children of sugar as such, or in sweets and cakes, should therefore be reduced to a minimum during the years of growth.

(v) The protein factor in the balance of diet should not be disproportionately increased through arbitrary addition to the diet of foods rich in protein such as meat, eggs and cheese, since a continued excess of it gives rise to severe disturbances of health.

(vi) The consumption of fat is also to be reduced to moderation, since a continued excess of fat disturbs the balance of the diet, with harmful consequences to health. Vegetable fats and butter from properly fed healthy cows are to be preferred to animal fats, since the latter contain poisonous metabolic waste products and are less easily digestible.

(vii) In a diet of full value, cooking salt should be used only in moderate quantities. In the goitrous districts of Switzerland the use of iodized cooking salt is recommended.

(viii) Fermented drinks of every kind containing alcohol should be completely excluded from children's diet.

(ix) Stimulants such as ground coffee, black tea, cocoa and chocolate—which furthermore are usually taken with refined sugar—are in no way beneficial to the growing child: their effect is only to excite the nervous system and the most delicate blood vessels. They deceive the nutritional instinct, which seeks to play its part in the sense of taste, and thus the instinctive regulation of the food balance is disturbed.

(x) Special mention should be made of the problem of the consumption of cow's milk in children's diet.
The differences in the composition of the milk of the mammal species reveal to us a performance of Nature which borders on the miraculous, and which—almost as if with foresight and wisdom—reckons up the correlations of all the various food factors for the needs of the sucking creature, and builds them up into its total diet.

The rate of growth of the creature, different with every species, determines the composition of the milk and the correlations of the food factors contained in it. Every species of mammal has therefore its specially compounded milk. Cow's milk is calculated to suit the speed of growth of the calf. The mother's milk of the human infant, whose rate of growth is slower, has a different composition from that of cow's milk, containing in particular considerably less protein. Because of this difference in composition and balance of factors, cow's milk, even if it is cleanly obtained from a properly fed cow, is an unsatisfactory substitute for the milk of the human mother. By diluting with water and mixing with lactose, or sugar of milk, an attempt is sometimes made to approximate its composition to that of human milk, which is incompletely successful. Even with the most careful artificial feeding on cow's milk, therefore, many infants show disorders of health.

From the second year onwards the growth of the child slows down more and more. Naturally feeding at the breast ceases, since the child's organism has meanwhile developed the tools—that is, the teeth—to deal with other foods. The milk has done its duty. The requirements of the organism have changed. The supply of iron which the new-born baby brought with it into the world, to last during the period of breast feeding, is now used up. In this respect, too, the milk, which contains no iron, can no longer suffice. Cow's milk has wrongly been recommended as a complete food for the child. The observations of children's doctors in regard to the nutritional effect of cow's milk upon the child have decided them to recommend from the second year onwards a prudent limitation in the quantity of it that is taken. With cow's milk as its sole food, even the two-year-old child would soon become sickly.

For the infant at this stage and for the older child, therefore, cow's milk is to be regarded only as a sparingly added supplement to its chief food—an average amount of ½ to ¾ pint per day is quite sufficient. Moreover the quality of the milk plays an important part. Its quality, as also its vitamin content, depends upon the feeding and on the condition of the cow. The best quality is obtained when the cow is at pasture. Cleanly obtained germ-free tuberculin-tested milk from healthy pasture-cows is the only kind of milk which can be taken unboiled, and may be unreservedly recommended for the diet of the child.

The ordinary untested milk should be taken only after it has been boiled. But the longer the action of the heat lasts upon it, the greater are the changes in its substance, and therewith the loss of its nutritive qualities.

According to Dr. Gerber the heat changes the following constituents of milk: the fat (change in power of cream formation), the lecithin (destroyed through splitting up of the phosphoric acid), the casein (changes its reaction to acid and rennet), the lactose (becomes caramelized), the citric acid (destroyed), the soluble calcium salts (transferred to an insoluble state), the carbonic acid (destroyed), the enzymes and vitamins (also destroyed). Great heat also destroys the bactericidal power of the milk.

All this applies chiefly to the sterilizing of milk, but it holds good in a lesser degree also for pasteurization. The usual domestic boiling stands, in its effect, somewhat between the two.

This aggregate of changes in the substance of cow's milk induced by heating, and not only the destruction of the vitamin C, makes it understandable why so many infants brought up on sterilized milk have lost their lives very painfully through Möller-Barlow's disease.

But it also teaches us that ordinary milk, boiled, is no very valuable item in the child's diet, and that the effort to obtain a "tested" milk that can be used unboiled for children's diet must be warmly greeted and supported.

Now that we have learnt what effects the heating of a single food, milk, has for its consequences in the substance itself and upon the health, the question logically follows: what effects and consequences for health is the influence of heat in our cookery able to produce upon all other foods?

(xi) Eggs: These foods, too, have suffered losses in quality and health value as a result of the incorrect feeding and various diseases of hens, and all manner of unreliable trading methods. As soon as eggs, even those of good quality, form a regular constituent of diet in any considerable quantity, they increase putrefaction in the bowels. We should therefore be very cautious about their use in children's diet.

The art of cookery has undoubtedly brought about a great enrichment of our table. Moreover, heat destroys bacteria and parasites (such as worm eggs and trichoniasis) which attach themselves to foods. Up till a short while ago it was even believed that heat burst open the vegetable cells which were enclosed by membranes, and thus rendered them susceptible to digestion. Through the researches bearing upon this point which were undertaken by Strasburger and Heupke it was, however, shown that such a supposition is not correct—indeed, the unboiled vegetable cells are turned to account by the digestive juices just as well as boiled ones.

The use of portions of animals' bodies in a raw state is confined in human diet to rare exceptions. In children's diet it does not need to be taken into consideration at all. The sense of taste refuses raw meat. It is the task of cookery to lend flesh food an agreeable taste. Furthermore, only heat is in a position to destroy the infection germs, tape-worm eggs and trichoniasis that may be contained in the meat. Cookery therefore entices mankind to the enjoyment of a material that has already been changed through the process of death, and further through heat, each involving a loss of nutritive values.

Our nutritional instinct and our taste behave in a very different manner towards the vegetable organisms which we use as foods. Enjoyment of them raw is felt to be natural, and the taste value richer and greater than if they were cooked. By proper manuring of the plants, and careful cleaning, the danger of infection and of worm eggs can be entirely avoided.

In spite of universal recognition of the advantages which it has conferred, the art of cooking has nevertheless, in so far as it prepares foods by heat, brought us many serious disadvantages for health, which have long escaped our recognition.

Forty years ago I made the surprising observation that well chosen and tastily prepared raw vegetable food is able to bring healing to very many widely spread disorders of health and serious diseases, in a quite astonishing fashion, where all other curative measures have failed. After protracted endeavours I found the solution of this puzzle. I recognized that the whole marvellous chemical structure of the living substance in the vegetable kingdom serves the purpose of a storehouse of sunlight, or rather of quanta of light from the sun's radiation, and that what nourishes both animal and human life is the sun's energy thus stored in the food. We are nourished not by calories, but by light quanta. Although I reached this conclusion along the road of the strictest scientific laws of energy, it was derided by contemporary authorities as unscientific, as mere mysticism and metagalaxis.* Not until 1934 was it brilliantly confirmed by the experimental researches of Crile, which showed that "the energy of the animal organism is supplied by a re-radiation of the sun's energy introduced into the body in vegetable foods," that, as Crile says, "the sun shines again in the proto-plasm of animals." The latter fact was given ocular demonstration by Crile.

This conclusion gave me the explanation of the heal-ing effect of raw food, and an indication for a biological and hygienic revaluation of foods and methods of pre-paring and dressing them up to the moment of serving at table. The formal chemical changes which the living substance undergoes until it becomes the finished food—that is, including the changes induced by heat—are the material expression of losses of energy. I thereby understood also the origin of so many diseases conveyed through cooked or otherwise degraded food.

Modern nutritional research has, step by step, brought corroboration of my ideas. Let me recall once more the serious illnesses of McCarrison's apes and of Stiner's guinea-pigs after eating cooked food. As soon as the investigators duly gave their animals raw food again they recovered. Recent research has shown that the vitamins, in particular vitamin C, are destroyed by heat where oxygen is present. Abelin of Berne concluded from the results of his own experiments that the protein substances, too, are damaged by heat.

I do not conclude from all this that the healthy man should live solely on raw vegetable food: only that raw vegetable food is the most potent healing factor that exists, and that it should form an essential constituent of human diet, and particularly of children's diet, as a protective food. Recent nutritional research has also

*Milk mush.—Tr.

come to exactly the same conclusion.

A diet which is composed solely, or mainly, of foods altered by heat (whether boiled, baked, roasted or sterilized), however plentiful and rich in protein, is in any circumstances a defective diet, from which illness will not be far absent. It is no longer open to question that heat upsets the balance of the food constituents and reduces the sunlight values of the diet.

The balance of the food constituents is also easily affected and disturbed by an excess of butcher's meat. The vegetable constituents also contain protein. The protein matter in green leaves is of great value, and is also better able to supplement the imperfect protein matter in seeds (such as grain, beans, lentils and peas) than is the protein in milk or meat. With a surplus of meat the protein content of the diet quickly becomes excessive, and so ill-balanced. Besides protein, meat further contains other substances which have a detrimental effect on health. In the course of time they produce the so-called supersensitiveness (allergy) out of which result abnormal reactions of the bodily vessels and all kinds of attacks, ultimately even high blood pressure.

It is constantly maintained by different writers that meat diet is necessary for mankind because its protein is superior to that contained in vegetables. I must contradict this assertion. Let the reader consider how many animals build up their entire bodies solely on vegetable protein.

In short, according to everything that I know and have observed during my life, animal meat of every kind does not on principle belong to children's diet. Children thrive better on a proper meatless diet, grow at a normal rate and display greater resistance to infection. Their strict observance of this practice is harmfully influenced, from an educational point of view, by the example of adults eating meat and the habit of associating plentiful helpings of meat with festal occasions.

I have still two questions to touch upon: (i) the question of quantity in diet and (ii) the question of the number of meals.

With wrongly balanced diet, the consequence is usually ravenous hunger in the child; but when the digestive organs refuse to function there is loss of appetite. Even the most plentiful of defective diets leads to eating too much and too often. The voracious appetite of the child is taken as a proof of a great need of food, which is thought to be in keeping with its rapid growth; and when she notices any lack of appetite the anxious mother presses an excess of food upon the child. Many children eat five times or more during the day, and in addition have sweets or chocolates between meals. The defective diet of our age has led to a lack of all moderation.

Long experience, no less than the nutritional experiments of the American physiologist Russel H. Chittenden, has taught us without any doubt that man thrives best on an economical provision of food such as just covers his need, and thus attains a higher capacity than with excessive feeding. This economical provision of food is only possible in the case of properly balanced diet, and on the assumption that it is thoroughly masticated.

With regard to the number of meals, let us remember that the Greeks of classical antiquity regarded a man who ate more than twice a day as a barbarian. The physiological process involved in the digestion of a full meal teaches us that the human organism would suffer no distress with only a single meal in the day. The organs which control the processes of digestion, no less than other organs, need their times of rest and regeneration. The same holds good for the organs of the child.

I have reached the conclusion that three meals a day, a chief meal and two frugal secondary meals, are not only sufficient, but also advantageous to health. All eating between meals, particularly of sweets, is prejudicial. "Elevenses" should be unconditionally abolished. If the "afternoon snack" must be retained, at least let the child be given nothing further than a piece of fruit and a small slice of wholemeal bread.

V

Food as nourishment and as stimulant and pleasure—

Preparation of raw and cooked foods

THE child requires food that is natural, and in no way over-refined. It requires the *whole* food, not artificially extracted food constituents.

1. FOODS EDIBLE IN THE NATURAL UNCOOKED STATE

Home-grown fruits: apples, pears, cherries, apricots, peaches, damsons, plums, grapes (not copper sulphate sprayed), figs, date-figs.*

Berries: strawberries, raspberries, bilberries, currants (red and black), blackberries, gooseberries, rose hips.

Southern fruits: oranges, mandarins, medlars, grapes, bananas, grapefruit, pomegranates, pineapples, lemons, melons.

Salads and leaf vegetables: cabbage lettuce, cos lettuce, spinach, dandelion, various cresses, chicory, endive, corn salad (or lamb's lettuce), beet spinach, purs-

*Known also as Japanese persimmon or "kaki".—TR.

lane, leeks, cabbages, savoy, white and red cabbage, fennel and the like.

Aromatic herbs: chive, parsley, marjoram, thyme, borage, tarragon, basil, summer savory, dill, mint, chervil, caraway and so on.

Roots: carrots, radishes (black and ordinary), beetroot, kohlrabi, celeriac, stacchys†, onions, garlic, etc.

Stalks and flower vegetables: rhubarb, celery, cauliflower.

Vegetable fruits: tomatoes, cucumbers, paprika pods (green) and so on.

Nuts: walnuts, hazelnuts, sweet almonds, brazil nuts, coconuts, pine kernels (but not peanuts or groundnuts‡).

Cow's milk only in the form of tuberculin-tested milk.

Important Rules: sweetening or salting?

No addition of sugar to fruit and berries: Both kinds of food contain rich quantities of the best sugar substance in harmonious balance with the other food factors. Addition of refined sugar upsets the natural balance and encourages the formation of acidosis. Refined sugar is not a product of Nature, not a natural whole food, but a technical preparation of extremely ill-balanced composition. The small child loves the sweetness that it so easily finds in sugar, and in no time its taste becomes accustomed to it. Now it wants only fruit with sugar added, and eats it thus even when there is no need for sweetening. In this way many children gradually lose their appetite for other foods. Out of anxiety their mothers give them still more sugared foods, instead of letting them go hungry until they gladly come

†Or Japanese artichoke.—Tᴿ.
‡Arachis: not strictly nuts at all, but pulses or legumes.—Tᴿ.

back to the natural unsweetened product out of hunger, and enjoy it. Sugar acidosis makes for poor blood, paleness and debility, and injures the growth of the bones and the teeth. So for preference never begin adding sugar to food! Getting rid of the sugar habit will come easily to a sensible person, if he makes an ally of hunger and himself sets an example to the child.

No addition of cooking salt to salads and raw vegetables: Salads and raw vegetables with green leaves, vegetable fruits, roots, stalks and flowers contain, besides their rich store of vitamins and other food factors, an abundance of the mineral substances which are important for life, in a natural harmonious balance and in serviceable form. They carry in themselves acid-forming as well as alkali-forming mineral substances, but the alkali-forming are always in preponderance. therefore these foods form, in conjunction with the fruits which have a similar preponderance of alkali, a reliable protection against the acidifying of the body, against acidosis. Because of this wealth of mineral substance the use of cooking salt is not only unnecessary, but it further alters the harmonious balance of the mineral substances in a manner detrimental to health.

Through discreet, knowledgeable use of the aromatic herbs and of onions such a high and agreeable taste value can be given to the preparation of salads and raw vegetables that even a fastidious palate does not miss the cooking salt.

On the preparation of salads, raw vegetables and fruit foods:

Two circumstances dictate the method of preparing these foods for serving at table: (i) long standing habits and refinement of taste, and (ii) diminished power and enjoyment of mastication, which is the consequence of innate or acquired dental weakness and dental disease. These circumstances are operative in a general way even in the case of children, if less noticeably than with adults, and moreover the attitude of the adult quickly colours that of the child.

A child with good strong teeth and natural hungry pleasure in mastication could, with advantage to its health, eat all these foods exactly as they come from the tree or the vegetable garden, after careful cleaning. Such a return to Nature is, however, as a general rule no more possible of achievement, nor is it desirable. Through preparation a great variety of nourishing, tasty, easily masticated foods can be obtained. French cookery knows many kinds of dishes made from raw vegetables under the name "hors d'oeuvres," though it often adds to them undesirable and unhealthy stimulants such as vinegar, mustard, pepper and salt.

The first process of preparation is cleaning. There are fruits and berries which require such cleaning. Apples and pears may be wiped over with a clean dry cloth. Berries should be picked over and, if necessary, washed in running water immediately before serving. Grapes, too, often require washing in this way. Dipping them in bowls of water at table is senseless.

For the cleaning of root vegetables no special directions are necessary, since in general this is done in the correct way. The cleaning of leaf salads and leaf vegetables, on the other hand, often leaves much to be desired. These extremely valuable foods are unfortunately all too often manured with liquid manure, which can spoil their taste and carries with it the danger of worm eggs. Anyone who is in a position to do so, should procure salads and vegetables from nurseries where organic (non-chemical) manure is used. In the kitchen the leaf vegetables and salads are put into a basin or a tub with plenty of water in which a small handful of cooking salt has been dissolved. After half an hour they are taken out and washed, leaf by leaf, in running water. In countries where there is known to be special danger of infection the leaves may be spread out in the sun, and each side exposed to its rays for a few minutes. If this is done after the washing, the water clinging to them must first be well shaken out. This shaking out is necessary in the case of all leaves which are to be eaten raw, e.g. in salads. If this method of cleaning is followed there need, in my experience, be no fear of worm infection.

The second process of preparation is the artificial chopping up of hard foods of this kind. This artificial chopping up serves two purposes: (i) the production of tasty dishes for the table which shall be pleasing to the eye, and (ii) the accommodation of raw vegetables to human chewing capacities.

Even among children the normal chewing capacity that mankind originally possessed is no more the rule. The universal diffusion of caries and pyorrhea among adults is symptomatic of a general constitutional deterioration which is passed on as a heritage to the children, so that the teeth do not possess their full hardness, or their proper enamelling, and all too often reveal abnormal formations, such as malocclusion,* which are prejudicial to good mastication. Soon children become subject to caries, as a consequence of their usually defective diet, whereby the chewing capacity undergoes a further weakening. The weaker the chewing capacity is, the more quickly arises the habit of swallowing insufficiently chewed mouthfuls of food, to the detriment not only of the digestive organs

*Failure of the teeth to articulate properly with their antagonists.—Tr.

but also of the utilization of the food.

The more defective the chewing capacity, and the further astray the habits of chewing from what they ought to be, the more necessary does artificial chopping up of food become. It may even be dispensed with altogether, in so far as it serves the second of the purposes mentioned above, where the child shows great chewing power and enjoyment of mastication, whether as an innate capacity or because under the influence of the diet here recommended the hardness of its teeth has gradually approached the normal, and the ability to masticate has been thus increased. Such a child will eat unchopped hard raw food with advantage to its teeth, for dental strength grows through the influence of harmonious diet from within, through the blood, as well as through practice. †

The chopping is done by a French knife‡, by grating into medium-sized or fine shreds, by fine slicing (e.g. cucumber), by cutting up small with a sharp knife (e.g. tomatoes), and by crushing with a pestle (e.g. berries). Berries, stoned cherries and plums may also be put through the mincer, as may dried fruits that have previously been softened in water, of which I shall speak later. The weaker the chewing capacity, the finer must the chopping of the hard food be. This holds good, for example, for celeriac, beetroot, carrots, white and red cabbage, kohlrabi and so on, which often require the finest shredding.

Even when chopped up in this manner, raw food still

†The same value that attaches to natural hard vegetables eaten raw is not to be ascribed to artificially hardened food, as for example hard bread or specially hardened crusts. No doubt such artificially hardened food can strengthen the teeth by giving them exercise. But the food content of hard bread and crusts has been depreciated by the excessive baking heat, and they should therefore not be given preference in children's food. Soft teeth can be damaged by such dry artificial hardness, where imperfect enamelling suffers small breakages in its surface.
‡Round two-handled chopping knife, which cuts with a rocking action.—Tr.

demands thorough mastication. There need be no fear that chewing capacity will be weakened through being thus spared some work by the chopping, as does happen in the case of boiled, soft or pulpy foods and white bread. The blood and the foundations of the teeth are better nourished by raw food, the teeth become hard again, and the chewing capacity increases.

The apple is a special case. Only the entire apple is a whole, an integral food. The throwing away of the peelings and the core involves a loss of food factors (vitamins and mineral substances) of high nutritional value, and at the same time a disturbance of the natural balance. For instance, the core contains twenty times as much iodine as the whole of the rest of the apple, a fact which in goitrous countries is of some importance. Even during my own childhood it was still reckoned a sin among the peasants not to eat the core of an apple. Today almost everyone peels the apple and removes the core, and confines himself to what remains of white apple flesh. Children copy their elders' example. Further, mistaken conceptions of medicine have spread the notion that peel and core are difficult to digest by reason of their rich cellulose content, and are thus dangerous for the digestive organs. This idea has today been proved to be entirely without foundation. A healthy child requires the whole apple, if it is to enjoy good health. The chief reason why most people no longer eat the whole apple, and so readily listen to false teaching on the subject, lies rather in the deplorable condition of the dental equipment of "civilized" man. Even in childhood the teeth become relatively soft through the customary methods of diet, and among 85 to 98 per cent of children of school age dental caries has already set in. If the adults who set the example are no longer able to masticate the whole apple properly, the children with their weak teeth also give up the attempt. How are we to make the eating of the whole fruit both possible and palatable for the children and adults of today?

It can be done simply by grating the apple, after removing the stalk and the calyx, into a mash. This should not be done until the moment before serving, as otherwise the mash will go brown through oxidization in the air. Apples thus mashed can be used for the production of a dish which will later be described, one which looks good and appetizing, and has strikingly beneficial results for the health of children and adults alike.

The third process of preparation consists in the addition of some binding nourishing substances to improve both the food value and the flavour—that is, in the provision of raw vegetable and fruit dishes for the table. With salads and chopped raw vegetables we mix salad dressing, for whose preparation the following food substances are used:

(i) vegetable oils: olive oil, nut oil, peanut or arachis oil and so on.

(ii) cream.

(iii) freshly squeezed lemon juice, or juices pressed from other fruits, cold-sterilized juice of fruit and grapes being also well suited for this purpose.

(iv) finely chopped aromatic herbs and onions.

Even the admixture of oil and lemon juice alone makes a very pleasant-tasting salad dressing. With a minimum of yolk of egg or nut cream, a mayonnaise can even be obtained from these two substances, which will tast excellent with tomatoes and shredded roots. The addition of aromatic herbs is a matter of taste, but is of not insignificant value for health. That onions have a high health value, and are furthermore thoroughly nourishing, should be well known. In the diet of the Bulgarians raw onions play a considerable part, and the relative rarity of cancer among the population of Bulgaria has been attributed to their plentiful use of onions as food.

In general I prefer raw extracted olive oil to all other oils, where food therapy is concerned; but the other oils are equally good food substances. Cream should be used only when the taste of the dressing needs moderating.

Bircher Muesli or raw fruit porridge

Chopped or grated fruit and mashed berries can be mixed with the following additions of other food substances to form fruit dishes which have proved their worth in children's diet:

(i) oatmeal, oat or Issroh flakes. For each helping of the fruit dish a single tablespoonful of oats should previously be soaked in two tablespoonfuls of water for twelve hours. When the apples become harder towards the end of winter, more water is needed.

(ii) freshly squeezed lemon juice. To each helping of the fruit dish is added the juice of half a lemon.

(iii) honey from the hive. To each helping one tablespoonful. To melt the honey, one pound of honey may be set in a basin of water, and warmed up with the addition of three tablespoonfuls of water until the right stage of fluidity is reached. The fluid honey easily mixes with the other constituents of the food.

Or else:

Sweet condensed milk. The presence in it of sugar is, certainly a disadvantage, but it makes possible the condensing and preserving of the milk at a temperature of only 131°F, whereby the natural food qualities of the milk are not injured. The advantage of mixing this condensed milk with fruit dishes is that it has a binding effect on the dish, the apple remaining a lovely white and being very agreeable to the palate. To every helping of the fruit dish is added one tablespoonful of sweet condensed milk.

The three ingredients so far mentioned are mixed together by stirring, and then one or two apples are immediately grated into them, or the fresh fruit or berry mash is added, and the whole is well mixed.

(iv) nuts, hazelnuts, sweet almonds, etc. To each helping of the fruit dish thus produced is added one tablespoonful of these (about ¾ oz.). If these kernels are finely milled in a nut mill, they may be sprinkled over the dish at table.

This fruit dish is the "muesli" which is already widely known in the world; from a health point of view it is an unsurpassed food for children, and may be given to any child from its second year onward—often it will even render good service to the infant during its first year, from the seventh month onward, especially in cases of sluggish bowels. (See recipe p. 61.)

For feverish diseases and digestive disorders among children, feeding with raw juices freshly pressed from fruit, berries and vegetables and different kinds of nuts (e.g. nut milk) is necessary. In cases of complete absence of appetite no food at all should be given for the time being. As soon as the demand for food makes its appearance, these juices should be the first and most important nourishment to be given. How this raw juice food, and particularly how the fresh vegetable juice dishes may be prepared, is described in the instructions contained in *Raw Fruits and Vegetables Book* (Keats Publishing). This liquid raw food has at the same time curative properties.

2. DRIED FRUITS AND DRIED VEGETABLES

Dried fruits of different kinds and dehydrated vegetables are the most natural, and from a health standpoint most acceptable, form of food preserves, and are surpassed only by the fruit and grape juices coldsterilized by the Seitz filtering process. Through being dried and stored they have lost certain food factors, and thus cannot in their nutritional effect be reckoned on a level with fresh foods, nor altogether take the place of these. For this reason these dried foods should be used in children's diet only in those gaps during the year when the supply of fresh foods is not sufficient. At such times they are undoubtedly a valuable form of nourishment. They should, however, not have been "beautified" by sulphurization!

Among dried fruits the following are well known: apple rings—for preference the kind that are dried in the old peasant fashion, skin, core and all—pears, prunes, cherries, apricots, plums, grapes, raisins, dates, bananas and pineapples.

By previous soaking in water for twelve to twenty-four hours, by stoning where necessary, and by putting through the mincer, they may be turned into a mash and also used for the making of "muesli."

Dried vegetables are little used. The best known are dried beans, but these are not suitable for eating raw, only for cooking. The Seitz "vegetable flours," however, are worthy of commendation. Among these are to be found, prepared by a skilful process, flour-like powders of dried parsley, young peas, aromatic herbs, lettuce, radishes, tomatoes, spinach, beetroot, green beans, celery, carrots and leeks. These "vegetable flours" can be eaten just as they are, dry, or mixed with fruit juices and olive oil. When there is no raw food to hand, or in certain cases of disease, they may render valuable service. It must naturally be understood that they need tasteful mixing.

3. BREAD

The most nourishing wholemeal bread would be yielded by freshly bruised grain (wheat, rye or a mixture of the two). During long periods of storage the food value gradually diminishes, the more quickly as the flour is more finely ground.

The often dirty, unnourishing outer husk of the grain is undesirable. Stefan Steinmetz has introduced a process of milling in which these husks of the fully grown corn are blown away by a stream of air, while the inner husk and the germ remain unharmed on the corn. There are said to be other milling processes, too, which are capable of achieving almost the same result.

It is not fine milling but the bruising of corn cleaned in this way, mixed with rye and wheat (in the proportion of 25 : 75) that provides the basis for the most nourishing possible bread, worthy to serve as the food of children, of the young generation with whom the future lies. The baking oven is not able to heat the inside of the bread beyond a temperature of 212°F., therefore the crumb of the bread is far more nourishing than the crust. Bread crust has been the subject of propaganda based on two incorrect assertions. Since roast products are present in it and its starch has been partially dextrinized, the taste finds it more attractive, which people confuse with "more nourishing." The roast products have hardly any food value, but excite the stomach glands to unnecessary discharge of their juices; yet the dextrine contains only a fragment of the food value of the starch from which it was formed. For that reason nutritional experiments also show that the nutritive and utilization value of crust is much smaller than that of crumb. The second assertion is that the greater the quantity and hardness of the crust, the more thoroughly it will need to be chewed, and so the healthier for the teeth. The supporters of this view are of the opinion that decay of the teeth springs from insufficient mastication. There is a certain modicum of truth in this opinion, but it has nothing to do with hard bread crust. Dental decay arises from the effect of defective and wrongly balanced diet upon the blood circulating in the pulp of the tooth, without regard to the hardness or softness of the food. Certainly the possessor of soft teeth, which are susceptible to disease, will incline towards soft food, since his pleasure in chewing has vanished. But hard bread crusts only make the blood worse, and so do no good to the teeth. Only a fundamental correction of the whole diet is capable of protecting and strengthening the teeth. On similar grounds Swedish hard bread ("crisp bread") cannot fulfil the promises that are made on its behalf.

All sorts of bread made from finely milled flour are unsuitable for children's diet: white bread, rolls, buns, biscuits, rusks, and especially the dextrinized wrongly so-called "invalids' bread." The flour from which they are baked is flour "milled to death." They no longer contain the vitamin and mineral substances of the grain, so that the body cannot use them to build up bone substance. The taking of such foods will with mathematical certainty destroy the balance of the diet. Rusks and "invalids' bread" are furthermore considerably devalued by the effect of a high degree of heat in their baking.

As a result of feeding on white bread and white flour products as their chief food, 4,000 workmen employed on the building of the Madeira—Marmoré railway in the neighbourhood of the Amazon died of beriberi.

Even if all the other constituents of the diet corresponded in every respect to the requirements of the laws of health, they would still be powerless to redress the balance in the struggle against the white flour products. Children will be exposed by such a diet to a hidden form of pre-beriberi.

Wholemeal bread needs a thorough exposure to salivary action through good mastication in the mouth. Children should therefore not crumble it into milk or coffee. Salivary action is the preparation for digestion in the stomach and the small intestine. It is therefore also to be recommended that this bread should, more often than is customary at present, be eaten dry and without any spreading of fat, since the fat impedes the action of the saliva.

Wholemeal bread needs no admixture of cooking salt, since it possesses in itself great richness of taste. In any case the use of cooking salt should be very sparing in all children's diet.

The baking process of wholemeal bread demands from the baker peculiar knowledge and care. When once the bulk of the population has grasped the immense significance of the transition from white bread to wholemeal bread for the health of coming generations, so that the bakers can supply this bread no longer as a speciality but as the normal product, its price will be able to be reduced below that of white bread. Every addition to the number of families who buy wholemeal bread for themselves and their children brings this time closer. No one should be put off by the somewhat higher price that is asked for it at the moment. Wholemeal bread is much more nutritious than white and a smaller quantity of it provides better nourishment than the customary amount of white bread, so that the yearly budget of a household will tip the scales in favour of the wholemeal.

4. COOKED VEGETABLES

Leaf, root and other vegetables. The cooking that is customary in most households destroys in leaf vegetables the greater part of the vitamin C whose working promotes the vigour of the biological processes, strengthens the walls of the blood vessels and prevents scurvy. The destruction begins even at a temperature of 140°F., and is the more serious the longer the cooking lasts. Spinach cooked in the customary fashion retains only a fortieth part of its original food content. We know that a relatively slight quantity of vitamin C in the whole diet is sufficient to prevent the onset of pronounced scurvy. This knowledge has led even doctors not to take its destruction in cooking seriously. But they are wrong. No one knows exactly how much vitamin C the human organism actually needs in order to remain in full health, but many observations and results of experiments suggest that a large number of serious injuries to health of a lingering character proceed from insufficient assimilation of vitamin C, even though the amount taken exceeds the theoretical "protective dose" against scurvy. Among the 341 children in Mooseheart this protective dose had to be increased more than five-fold, to bring to an end the subtle injuries that were occurring to their gums and teeth.

This is one of the most serious grounds for my insisting, in agreement with all nutritional investigators of standing, that in a healthy diet raw vegetables as well as cooked ones should always be present as an essential constituent. If this requirement is fulfilled in children's diet, good supplementary nutritional effects may also be expected from vegetables sensibly cooked.

Spinach, for instance, we cook in the following way: half the quantity to be cooked of some tender spinach is brought for only a single instant to the boil in thin vegetable stock,* then chopped up small. The other half is chopped up raw. Then onions are fried to a light brown colour in butter, mixed with a little flour, and added to the boiled bulk of spinach. Then the whole is thinned with some of the spinach water that is left over, and boiled for about half a minute. Lastly the raw spinach is added to it in the pan, and as soon as the whole comes to the boil after some half a minute to a minute, the vegetable is ready for serving.

Our aim should be wherever possible to shorten the time of cooking and so to attain an even higher degree of relish in the taste. If at all possible, the nutrients present in the vegetables should persist when these are cooked. Therefore one should, so far as one can, avoid pouring away the water in which they are boiled, and where this is not possible the water should be used for soups or as an addition to other dishes.

This type of cooking differs fundamentally from the French method, which pours away the water in which vegetables are boiled, together with the vitamins and mineral substances contained in it (i.e. the vegetables are scalded). It is this latter method which is used in hotels and the majority of hospital kitchens. The natural taste of the vegetables is thus for the most part lost. To cover up their tastelessness, meat broths, extracts and meat sauces are then added to them, so that often the most various vegetables finish up with the same unnatural taste. Even in the medical literature of our own day we find directions to blanch spinach twice

*The Bircher-Benner Clinic suggests that this stock can be replaced by a broth made from Marmite or other yeast extract, with Vecon (vegetable extract), obtainable at health food stores.—Tr.

51

for disorders of the stomach. All the evidence of research teaches us that such a method of cooking is injurious to health. Our method strives to preserve the food value of the vegetables; it is conservative.

The effect of boiling and steaming upon whole potatoes is less harmful. They are to some extent protected by their skin from loss of mineral substances, and their bulk protects the insides against the permeation of the heat. Young, still unripe potatoes and old seed potatoes should not be eaten raw, as then their relatively high solanine content might be injurious. The potato is therefore worthy of special commendation as a cooking vegetable. The best method of cooking potatoes is to roast them whole or halved, skin and all, in the oven on a buttered tin. In the case of halved potatoes the cut surface may be pressed on to some caraway seeds,* and the vegetable then put into the oven with the seeds sticking to it, facing downwards on the tin. Children are particularly fond of potatoes prepared in this way.

A feature of quite irreplaceable value in a healthy cookery method is the vegetable stock† which is everywhere taking the place of meat stock, and appears in all soups. Directions for making it, and many other suggestions besides, as well as menus for a whole year's meals, are to be found in *Health-giving Dishes* by Frau Bertha Brupbacher-Bircher (Edward Arnold).

5. CEREALS

Whole-grain buckwheat, buckwheat porridge or flakes;

Coarse or pot barley, fine pearl barley, barley flakes or flour;

---

*Or other herbs or seeds.—TR.
† See p. 51 note—TR.

Whole "Greencorn," as porridge, flakes or flour;
Whole-grain oats, oatmeal, porridge or flakes;
Whole-grain millet, millet flakes;
Maize (Indian corn), maize porridge or flour;
Rice (brown, unpolished), rice (white, unpolished with remnants of silvery skin), polished rice, rice flakes or flour;
Whole-grain rye, rye flakes or flour;
Sago, tapioca;
Whole-grain wheat, whole-grain semolina, ordinary semolina, wheat flakes, wholemeal flour, plain flours,* fine white flours;
Wheat-germ in the form of small flakes.

6. PULSES (AS SUPPLEMENTARY ALTERNATIVES TO CEREALS)

Haricot beans, white, fresh or dried;
Peas, fresh or dried, split or milled;
Flageolet beans, dried;
Lentils, whole, shelled or milled;
Chestnuts, fresh, dried or milled;
Soya bean flour.

The cereals and pulses here enumerated complete the dietary for children. The flour products (cereals in milled form) should, however, not be used for soups and other dishes; use instead, as far as possible, the grain or porridge forms that have first or second place in the above list. When grain is used in this way it should be previously soaked in cold water all night, and then cooked the next day in the same water, and served as soup or broth. (See Frau Bertha Brupbacher-Bircher's cookery book for a great variety of recipes.) Health food stores supply all pulses and cereals not obtainable at the ordinary grocers.

---

*Stone-ground plain flour, containing part of the wheat germ, is obtainable at health food stores.—TR.

7. FOODS FROM THE RANGE OF HUMAN DIETRY WHICH SHOULD NEVER, OR ONLY EXCEPTIONALLY, BE GIVEN TO THE CHILD

I know that my decision to exclude the following foods will by no means be met with general agreement. But I am not writing for those who are of another opinion, I am writing because after long experience and much research my medical conscience bids me do so. Those who attend to me will not regret it.

From children's diet we should exclude:

Flesh foods: that is to say, every kind of meat from slaughtered animals, birds, fish and molluscs. I exclude this form of food not because of being a vegetarian, but as a doctor. The grounds for my verdict may be discovered in my writings, and partly also in my introductory remarks. The consequences of years of meat diet for human health are much more serious than is realized even by the average doctor. The eating of meat also becomes a confirmed habit, the breaking of which is not easy. Therefore better not begin it. In addition, the harm done by meat during the years of growth is more serious than in the case of adults.

Meat broths and all meat extracts.

All fermented alcoholic drinks.

White bread, rolls and rusks should be exceptions only.

Refined white sugar, and also other sugar extracts taken with food and drink in the form of sweets or sweet cakes with finely milled flour should be given to children only exceptionally—say, on festal occasions.

Tinned preserves: these foods sterilized by heat are dead food, whose food factors have been largely damaged. Let us remember the illnesses of McCarrison's apes and Stiner's guinea-pigs. Even if according to the animal physiologist Scheunert, who puts in a good word for preserves, all preserve factories produced their wares in conditions which excluded oxygen, and thus retained the vitamin C—which is certainly not the case—so many other changes of substance would still occur in the preserved products that they would have to be reckoned as defective foods. Therefore these preserves are not suited to the normal diet of children. Only in case of need are they permissible, for they are certainly better than nothing. This conclusion applies with almost equal force to home bottled preserves. They, too, are only emergency foods.

Jams and candied fruits: with these foods there is not only the change induced by heat to be considered, but also the strong increase of the sugar content, which serves to make them an undesirable influence upon the health of the child's body. Therefore I must warn my readers against regular, or even frequent, eating by children of these artificial products.

Chocolate contains a stimulant to the nerves and other vessels of the body, and a strong admixture of sugar. All assertions concerning its high food value, as in advertisements, are not to be taken seriously. Bodies injured by chocolate are difficult to heal. The eating of it should not be allowed to become a habit with children.

Coffee and tea are also superstimulating to the nervous and vascular system, and in no way promote health. They should play no part in the regular diet of the child.

Among the bulk of children in whose diet the foods and stimulants here excluded are taken regularly and in considerable quantities, a premature lankiness of growth makes its appearance, and often an abnormal rise in the temperature of the body, and early decay of the teeth; further, such children also show an increased susceptibility to disease of all kinds.

The diet here recommended for children is simple and frugal, but it has quality. My own seven children have been brought up on such a diet. One need not be well-to-do in order to feed children in this way. The parent who is compelled by an insufficiency of worldly goods to give his children but little meat and sweets, need no longer feel jealous of the rich who are better provided for. It is just the rich who have to pay a heavy price for their luxury diet and the faulty feeding which they do not recognize as such, in the form of the illnesses and pains which sooner or later overtake their children. Dr. Paul Carton, a French doctor, has pointed out how, with the increase of prosperity, serious illnesses have made their appearance, through "improvements" in diet from generation to generation.

Children require a natural, whole and non-artificial diet, a diet which God and Nature and the living principle have compounded and created. These wonderful, harmoniously attuned atomic and molecular structures, charged with light, these never fully fathomable eternal riddles of chemistry, these formations of air, water, light, life and spirit—these are designed for us men as food. Should not reverence prevent us from changing them arbitrarily and thoughtlessly before we incorporate them in our bodies? We cannot ourselves build up even the smallest of them, but we can and do tear them to pieces and destroy them. Only we have not considered that in so doing we are also tearing to pieces and destroying by a lingering process the bodies, the bones, the teeth and the blood of our children, the coming generation of mankind, and setting an insulating layer that becomes increasingly thicker between the life that is within us and the Spirit.

The decline of the West begins in the physiological sphere, in the degeneration of the diet of civilized nations. Social misery, spiritless politics and mutual exacerbation are only the biological consequences of our physiological perversity. The great seer Nietzsche rightly says of the consequences of the meals which people take nowadays: "and whatever they may do, pepper, ill-temper or world-weariness will control their conduct!" And in another place he says: "It is through complete lack of sense in the kitchen that man's development has been longest retarded and worst impaired."

For forty years I have been observing the effects of diet upon the human body and soul among many thousands of invalids, and hundreds of careful and reliable investigators have helped me with the results of their researches, to penetrate the connections between diet and disease, diet and health. Thousands have found health again through food therapy which I have prescribed. I can see how the much extolled diet of the civilized nations is gnawing like a worm at the very marrow of humanity. The mischief is moving forward with rapid strides. In this vitally important question our leading men and women are ignorant; biased and dazzled by vested interest, they do not see what is ahead of them. But mothers and fathers who love their children would do well to think over what I am saying, and when they understand it, go boldly and fearlessly to work to correct their children's diet.

8. THE CHILD'S MEALS

Infants (6-12 months)	Babies (from 1-2 years)	Toddlers (over 2 years) and older children

Breakfast, between 6.0 and 8.0 a.m.

7-9 oz. of mother's milk or	1 ripe fruit cut up small or	1 plate of muesli, or 1 or 2 apples or cit-

57

Infants (6-12 months)	Babies (from 1-2 years)	Toddlers (over 2 years) and older children

Breakfast, continued

5-5½ oz. of cow's milk with 3½ oz. of gruel, or 9 oz. of nut milk* with gruel and the necessary fruit juices.	1 small bowl of ripe berries or stone fruit mashed or chopped with 1 cup of unboiled, perhaps slightly warmed tuberculin-tested milk (perhaps with some gruel), and 1 crust of wholemeal bread (later on, one slice).	rus fruit (or stone fruit or berries) with 1 cup unboiled tuberculin-tested milk, and 1 or 2 thick slices of wholemeal bread, with or without butter (ordinary or nut).

Dinner, between 11.0 a.m. and 1.0 p.m.

Vegetable purée (see recipe) pressed through a sieve, 7-9 oz.	Vegetable stew (see recipe), either mashed with a fork or left as it is.	Some raw fruit; perhaps cereal soup or vegetable soup; perhaps one cooked vegetable, 2 or 3 kinds of raw vegetables as salads; in addition a potato or egg dish.

Tea, between 3.0 and 4.0 p.m.

7 oz. of mother's milk or 7-9 oz. cow's milk or nut milk thinned down with gruel, perhaps also a small crust of bread.	1 small plate of raw vegetables with lemon juice, oil or cream (see recipe).	Fruit; if necessary, 1 slice of bread, spread with cottage cheese.

*Diluted nut butter (health food stores)

Supper, between 6.0 and 7.0 p.m.

| 7 oz. of finest muesli (see recipe); if still breast-fed, more mother's milk may follow later. | Muesli of a coarser kind (see recipe), perhaps 1 slice of wholemeal bread. | Ordinary muesli with whole nut kernels (including almonds) perhaps a small additional warm dish (soup or potatoes), or wholemeal bread and 1 cup of milk (varying according to season and individual need). |

9. RECIPES

Vegetable Puree for babies

Bring a pint of water to the boil, and stir in two heaped teaspoonfuls of cereal (preferably in the form given second in the list on pages 52-3). Avoid oats, since these are used daily for muesli, also any cereal which has already figured the same day in the infant's gruel. If crusts are given, coarse wheat may be occasionally left out for the sake of change. Once a week at this age, pulses (preferably split lentils) may take the place of cereals. One teaspoonful of soya flour, mixed with water and boiled up with cereals, makes a suitable addition two or three times a week.

When water and cereals have boiled for a few minutes, add a medium-sized, unpeeled, well scrubbed potato, cut into pieces, and also 1½-3 oz. of vegetables, well cleaned and cut up small. Suitable vegetables for children under a year old are young carrots or other roots, cauliflower, salsify, celery, kohlrabi, fennel, spinach (not manured), lettuce, Romaine or cooking lettuce, endive and Japanese artichokes. On the other hand, peas, beans and Brussels sprouts should be given sparingly, and added to other vegetables. Cabbage should be reserved until the child is older.

When vegetables and potatoes are tender (about 20 minutes), the whole stew is passed through a sieve and a small quantity of butter (about the size of a hazel nut) is added.

In order to ensure a proper supply of vitamins, every other day the sieved pulp of a small ripe tomato or a tablespoonful of carrot juice, according to season, should be added to the stew when finished. The latter may easily and quickly be obtained by grating one or two carrots (preferably on a two-way grater) and pressing them through a fine sieve (preferably hair), by crushing and kneading with a wooden pestle or squeezing them through muslin until sufficient juice has been obtained. In the end, the finished stew should weigh 7-8 oz. No salt should be added and sugar only if the child refuses the dish unsweetened.

Vegetable Stew for toddlers

This may be made according to the recipe given above, only in rather larger quantities. At first it should be mashed only with a fork, if at all; and later it is served as it comes from the saucepan. It may be slightly salted, and carrot juice or tomato pulp may be dispensed with, as the child should now be having a small amount of proper raw vegetable salad. Instead, two or three times a week, on days when no soya flour is used, the yolk of an absolutely fresh egg may be added to the stew when finished.

First attempts at raw vegetables for small toddlers

Cleaned carrots are grated on a really fine grater (e.g.

a nutmeg grater), and sprinkled with lemon juice, oil or cream.

Or

A few nice light-green lettuce leaves, or a handful of corn salad (lamb's lettuce) or endive, or chicory leaves are cut up small, and sprinkled with a little lemon juice and some oil.

Or

A fully ripe tomato is washed, cut up, and crushed with a fork, then mixed as before with lemon juice, oil or cream.

Before long this raw diet may be widened to include grated radish, celery, kohlrabi, a little spinach (unmanured), cress, etc.

Muesli

1. For babies up to one year.

A heaped teaspoon of finest oatmeal (or other fine flakes by way of a change) is soaked in two tablespoon-densed milk, add a little nut butter (the tip of a spoonful), procurable at health food stores; and stir well in a bowl. Keep stirring, and gradually add the soaked flakes, together with a few drops of lemon juice. Then halve a medium-sized apple, quickly grate it after removing core (the skin remains on the grater), stir it into the mixture and serve immediately. According to season, the juice of half an orange or a tablespoonful of bilberries or raspberries, grapes or wild strawberries pressed through a sieve, may be added to the muesli. This dish is an ideal substitute for milk puddings or porridge.

2. For babies and toddlers 1-2 years.

Soak a tablespoonful of fine flakes in cold water. In winter these should if possible be mixed with wheatgerm for their rich vitamin content. Add a little lemon juice and a tablespoonful of condensed milk or liquid honey, then a good-sized apple grated on a fine (preferably two-way) grater, skin and all. Grated nuts of as many different kinds as possible should be sprinkled over the muesli, which is then served immediately. Instead of apples, other kinds of fruit or berries may be used, crushed with a fork. (N.B. Strawberries are often found not to agree with very small children.)

3. *For toddlers and older children.*

If the child can chew well, the recipe for adults (see page 44) may be followed. In place of grated nuts sprinkled over the dish, use whole nut kernels of various kinds.

Gruel for thinning cow's milk or nut milk

Two tablespoonfuls of cereals are soaked overnight in 2 pints of water. In the morning they are boiled in the same water for half an hour, until half the water has evaporated. If the gruel is to be sweetened, boil a heaped teaspoonful of brown (preferably cane) sugar with it. Rice gruel should be used only for children with a tendency to diarrhea.

For cow's milk, see page 29.

As a drink, in addition to the fresh fruit juices, rose-hip tea is particularly to be recommended, on account of the remarkable richness of its vitamin C content. Rose-hip pips and pulp are previously soaked for 24 hours in cold water, then boiled in the water for half an hour, and sweetened with a little brown (preferably cane) sugar. Drunk warm, the tea tastes excellent; it is also tasty and refreshing if taken cold, with a few drops of lemon juice added to it. (Rose-hip puree, as a jam, is preferable to all other sweet spreads.)

VI

Examples of the effect of nutrition in experiment and medical experience

OF the many examples known to me I shall give here only a small selection. Some of them concern dental diseases which, as we now at length realize, are always a sign that the other organs and tissues of the whole body are also under the sway of disease, and that the diet is at fault. Through a correction in the errors of diet and through the achievement of balance in its composition, the course of the dental diseases can be brought to a standstill. This successful result is a proof of the real nutritive value and the suitability of such curative feeding for human needs. But at the same time it gives us an indication how to avoid these diseases by corrections of our diet that correspond to those needs. We must not forget that the healing diet which checks, or even cures, the dental diseases at the same time frees the remaining organs and tissues from the pressure of disease.

1. THE EFFECT UPON GUINEA-PIGS OF FOOD COOKED BY STEAM PRESSURE

Guinea-pigs exposed to a lack of vitamin C display

the same sensitiveness as human beings, Dr. O. Stiner, an investigator of the Swiss Board of Health in Berne, gave a large group of guinea-pigs their normal food, which they otherwise took raw (oats, hay, carrots and water), cooked in a high-pressure steamer. By this treatment the vitamin C was destroyed and numerous other changes in the food substances, of which nothing more exact is at present known, were brought about.

These guinea-pigs fell victims to softening of the teeth to such an extent that the teeth could be cut away with scissors. Gangrenous gingivitis followed, and a softening of the jaw bones induced a warping tendency in the jaw, so that the rows of teeth overlapped and would not close properly. The gums grew scorbutic, and the salivary glands diseased. The effect of this feeding on the remaining tissues and organs of the body was made obvious by the fact that the animals became anemic, got goiter, and finally succumbed to scurvy and to some extent to cancer of the lung. When Stiner added 10 c.c. (about two teaspoonfuls) daily of pasteurized milk to these animals' food, a serious disease of the joints, arthritis deformans, made its appearance.

2. THE EFFECT OF TEN DAYS' EXCESSIVE MEAT DIET

In the University Hospital at Tübingen Dr. Otfried Müller has introduced the new research method of microscopic histology of the capillaries, which is of the highest significance for the investigation of human health. Even with a magnification of 60 the eye sees in the skin through the horny layer or in the mucous membrane of the lips the fine hairpin-like loops of the smallest blood vessels which exist in the human body, to the number of about five thousand million. These capillaries are, so to say, the trade ports and trans-shipping stations of the tissues and organs for the receiving of nourishment and disposal of waste products. If their condition deteriorates, the nourishing and cleansing process of the tissues deteriorates also. By means of microscopic examination the eye also sees the streaming blood and is able to observe the speed of its flow. Under the influence of the quality of the diet the blood that flows through the capillaries changes, and this change is reflected in the condition of the capillaries. Certain parts of the capillary system are peculiarly sensitive to changes in the blood as a result of injurious diet, for example those of the gums and pulp of the teeth. Capillary damage invariably signifies some damage to the whole body.

Professor Gänsslen, the colleague of Otfried Müller, made the following observations by means of capillary microscopy in a nutritional experiment on two young students. Their "capillary pictures" were photographically recorded; they looked normal. Each of them was then given, over a period of ten days, a daily diet of 1500 g. (about 3 lbs.) of meat of all kinds in wide variety, together with 30 g. (about 1 oz.) of white bread and lemonade. At the end of ten days their capillary pictures were again recorded. Result: the capillaries had swollen into broad elongated bags, ruptured in places by blood diffusing out into the surrounding tissue. The blood stream was slowed down, and the blood itself congested.

While both of them had taken the experimental diet willingly and without any resistance or complaint, at the end of this short experimental period a scorbutic swelling of the gums set in, so that they bled easily, and the young men's skin had strikingly reddened—as Gänssler says, it was like a butcher's skin.

A meatless diet of over a month's duration was needed to bring about a gradual return of the capillaries to their normal condition.

Thus, in the short operative period of only ten days, one-sided meat diet had appreciably damaged the most intimate and vital structures of the youthful body, the very marrow of the organism, and with it the organs and tissues. What one-sided meat diet manages in ten days, regular meat diet will see to in twenty or thirty years.

3. DR. BIENSTOCK'S HIGH BLOOD PRESSURE

At the age of thirty-three this doctor's health began to weaken. He consulted numerous authorities, and had himself thoroughly examined in hospital. Kidney trouble was found, but the cause of the disease was not revealed. Finally a series of attacks of blindness and general decrepitude made their appearance, together with raised blood pressure. After more than thirty years of suffering he returned, completely enfeebled, to a university hospital. After the examination the professor let him go, as ill as he had come, with the advice in his extremely weak condition not to deviate from his meat diet. In the despair that now seized him he made up his mind on his own responsibility to renounce completely every form of animal protein. And behold, from that same day all the serious symptoms of disease, even the attacks of blindness, began to decline, and the strength of this sixty-seven year-old man gradually returned to him.

This puzzling experience gave the doctor the idea that through the taking of meat, cheese, eggs and milk from his childhood onward, there had quite gradually arisen in his body a supersensitiveness, or allergy, towards animal protein, so that he owed his protracted sufferings to these foods. He decided to put the matter to the test. On the first occasion he ate a helping of egg noodles. On the following day came a new attack of illness, which, however, quickly yielded to a further abstinence from animal protein. Then he ate quite a small piece of ham. Result: a serious attack of illness, with clouding of the vitreous humour in the eye. Further systematic attempts established his hypersensitiveness to animal protein even in quite small quantities.

Bienstock now described his illness and his observations in a professional medical journal, and closed with the conclusion that he had drawn: "My high blood pressure with all its attendant phenomena and symptoms is an allergic animal-protein poisoning; might not a similar cause be assigned to the cases of the many millions of other human beings with this disease?"

Dr. Bienstock's suggestion may be endorsed. I have myself seen many invalids with high blood pressure get well again after correction of their diet by an exclusion of meat.

But this experience shows the total blindness which prevailed in medical circles, and still prevails, with regard to the effects of animal foods, and particularly of meat, upon the human organism. A man who was a doctor suffered for thirty-three years, and consulted every authority. Not one of them had even the faintest inkling of the causal connection of the disease, nor was the advice they gave of the slightest value.

Let parents reflect that if they accustom their children to meat diet, they are laying the foundations for allergic animal-protein poisoning in later years, with all its grave consequences.

4. DR. WILLIAM HOWARD HAY'S KIDNEY DISEASE

The American surgeon Dr. Hay fell a victim towards the end of his thirtieth year to chronic inflammation of the kidneys. According to his university-gained knowledge he was a lost man. His science knew of no means of healing this disease; it was held to be incurable. In despair he went his own way: he changed his diet. His solution was never to eat unless he was hungry, and then only natural foods of vegetable origin. And in this way Dr. Hay became well again! But now his notions of medical treatment underwent a change. His experience had taught him that the composition of a diet is of decisive importance for health and for recovery from disease, and it had further shown that his science knew nothing at all about this connection and about such methods of therapy.

He plunged into the problem of diet, and began to prescribe fundamental correction of diet for those invalids who found no recovery through the customary treatment; in so doing he achieved the most wonderfully successful cures. He now founded at his home a large sanatorium, in which numbers of invalids recovered their health. He reported upon his experiences in his book, *A New Health Era*.

"But," says Dr. Hay, "we keep to a perverted diet until one is seriously ill, why not begin by correcting children's diet so that they never become ill?"

5. DR. BOITEL'S REPORT UPON THE ORPHAN CHILDREN OF VEVEY

In Vevey on the Lake of Geneva there is a private orphanage, which on extremely limited means accepts the children of destitute parents or helpless orphans and maintains and educates them. Thanks to an excellent management the children are accustomed to a sound regimen and a very simple, almost meatless diet. They see to it that the children never eat between meals, or just before a meal. Sweets are almost entirely barred. For breakfast the children have a kind of Bircher "muesli."

The school dental clinic in the town of Vevey superintends the condition and repair of the teeth in the orphanage, as well as in the State schools. The school dentist, Dr. Boitel, reports as follows:

"It is a fact well known to the school dental clinic that the girls from the orphanage have good teeth. During the past eight years we have found with these children, on the first examination, an average of 3.5 carious cavities per child, and from the second to the seventh years of their stay in the orphanage onwards, 1.3 cavities per child, .02 treatments of the roots of teeth were carried out per child, and not one single extraction. During the same period of observation we found among the other school children of the city an average of 3.8 cavities per child per year.

"On entering the orphanage the children had no better teeth than the average. During the whole period of their stay there they only had a third of the amount of caries that other children of the town showed. And not only that, but the teeth are finer; they impress one by their cleanness, their healthy colour, and by the normal condition of the gums."

6. DR. MONTIGEL OF CHUR REPORTS UPON HEALTHY TEETH IN AN ORPHANAGE

In the Swiss Canton of Graubünden there is an orphanage with its main buildings in Zizers and three branches in other villages, which takes in deserted, poor children, rather below the average of health, from infancy onwards, and educates them up to school-leaving age. The wards of this institution are distinguished by their healthy teeth. While in the upper-class environment of the Chur* School, in the first class only 1 to 3 per cent of the children are free from caries,

*Capital of the Canton.—Tr.

"the Ruflins (orphanage) children show on their entrance to school half of them faultless teeth, and on the average of their whole number we find, on a first examination, 23.9 per cent of all the children free from caries.

"Everyone who understands the subject knows that this state of things is far above the normal level for Switzerland."

Now let us see what the diet of these children is. Dr. Montigel speaks of it as follows:

"The Zizers institutions draw from their own farms what they need in the way of milk, vegetables and fruit. They sell only the surplus, keeping back abundant supplies for their own households. Bread has recently been improved through home baking. But the consumption of bread is not large, since the children eat it only at their afternoon snack (of fruit and bread) and occasionally at night. In the place of bread, for breakfast they have oatmeal porridge, cooked throughout the night in self-cookers, which forms the sole breakfast of the children. The daily ration of oatmeal for the Zizers households consists of 19 lbs. The whole institution contains some sixty-five children and thirty adults, so that this works out at about 3 oz. a head. The children eat meat only on special festal occasions, the adults on Sundays in addition.

"If we survey the diet that is carried out at Zizers it is evident that it broadly corresponds with modern dietetic principles. . . . For the small children fresh fruit every day, for the older ones similarly fresh fruit or uncooked dried fruit daily. For all the inmates, from the earliest ages upwards, green vegetables daily. On this form of diet the children feel extraordinarily well. Their fresh healthy colour, the statistics of their weight, the slight incidence of disease among them, above all, too, the condition (far above the average) of their teeth, are a proof that the diet is good and appropriate in every direction."

These orphan children with their simple diet are thus far better cared for than the town children, and even than the country children, of Switzerland.

7. RESULTS OF EXPERIMENTS BY BUNTING, HADLEY, JAY AND HART

These four American investigators have followed in five groups, varying in number between 74 and 159 children, the effects of the care of teeth, with and without corrected diet, over a long period of observation. They sum up their conclusions as follows: "Among the three groups who were given a properly combined diet, consisting primarily of milk, fruits and vegetables, dental decay became increasingly rare, or was altogether prevented. Among the other groups, with a diet which—although it was in the usual sense plentiful and "good"—did not satisfy the requirements of recent nutritional teaching, the dental decay could not be checked in spite of antiseptic cleaning of the teeth, and the disease quickly got the upper hand."

8. THE 341 CHILDREN OF THE CHILD COLONY AT MOOSEHEART IN ILLINOIS, U.S.A.

Diet and Dental Health is the title of a book in which Milton T. Hanke, the scientific director of investigations carried out by a group of thirteen dentists, gives a report upon their progress and conclusions.

This group of investigators had come to realize that the slight inflammation of the gums which is so very widespread, although not a serious condition, was nevertheless a sign of disordered health in the whole body, from which the gravest consequences could spring. "We can observe the changes which reveal themselves in the mouth, but not the changes which occur at other points in the body," as they expressively put it.

They observed on the teeth themselves, simultaneously with the onset of the inflammation of the gums, little patches of different colour in the enamel of the teeth. They were able to establish the fact that these patches arise through a local decalcification,* and that it was in these places that caries later on began. They concluded that caries, too, starts from within, as does inflammation of the gums, and that, like the latter, it is a sign of internal disorders of health, which have also affected other parts of the body.

The investigators were thus convinced that the appearances in the gum and the enamel of the tooth, as indicating a general sickening in the body, might be interpreted as pre-scorbutic symptoms. But for scurvy the citrus fruits, oranges and lemons, are pre-eminently suited as a means of cure. So the question they set themselves to answer in their great experiment was: what effect have the citrus fruits upon the diseased gums and the teeth?

Mooseheart is an educational settlement on the Fox River, for the care of children between the ages of ten and seventeen, under favourable climatic and country conditions, and distinguished educational and medical direction. It contains on the average some 1,200 children who form in several houses families of about fifteen apiece. The diet is better than the average in America, but in spite of this fact inflammation of the gums and dental caries show a high frequency among the children.

This children's colony now placed itself at the dis-

*Weakening of the lime.—Tr.

posal of the investigators. Three hundred and forty-one children were chosen and observed over a period of three and a half years. For the first year nothing in their customary regimen was altered, but the incidence of inflammation of the gums and dental caries were precisely noted. During the whole of the second year, each of the children was given daily a pint of orange juice and the juice of a lemon, whereat the reaction of the gums and the teeth was established. In the third year the first year's regimen was again instituted, only the children were given an average of 3 fluid oz. of orange juice every day—the amount known to be the "protective dose" against scurvy.

The conclusions of this wide-scale nutritional experiment were stated thus: "The addition of a pint of orange juice and the juice of one lemon to the daily diet leads to an almost complete disappearance of the gingivitis, a 50 per cent reduction in the incidence of dental caries, and a marked increase in the rate of growth.

"Dental caries again becomes rampant and gingivitis redevelops in most of the cases when the citrus fruit intake is reduced to three ounces a day for one year. Three ounces is not enough."

So the scurvy protective dose is not enough!

It should be noted that in these experiments no general correction of the diet was undertaken. A fundamental correction of the whole diet, in the sense which I have advocated in this booklet, would have brought about at least an equal success. This is important to realize, since it is impossible to guard the children of the whole world against illness by giving each of them a pint of orange juice and the juice of a lemon every day of their lives. But the great significance of certain constituents of a diet is brilliantly demonstrated by the Mooseheart experiment.

9. THE CURE OF AN OTHERWISE INCURABLE DISEASE BY RAW VEGETABLE DIET

The Herter-Heubner* disease is a very serious children's disease which manifests itself in retarded growth and serious symptoms in the intestinal tract. The children display swollen bellies, bulky faces, and waste gradually away in spite of every care and previous treatment. Pronounced cases used to be considered incurable. But in my opinion there is definitely a frequent occurrence of less pronounced cases among children, which in the course of time somehow get better "of their own accord."

The six-year-old Lala M. was, when she came to me for treatment, a pronounced case. She only weighed 24 lbs. Long medical treatment in a high mountain district and five months' treatment in the Zürich children's hospital had done little for her. Nobody had dared, in the precarious condition of her digestive organs, to give her anything raw to eat, even an apple. In despair her mother asked me to undertake the treatment of the child.

This seriously diseased child recovered within eight months by means of an exclusive suitably prepared diet of raw fruit and vegetables, supported by heliotherapy and hydrotherapy. She increased 15¼ lbs. in weight during this time, and grew 2¾ inches in height.

Since this cure of Lala M. the children's hospital at Zürich has introduced a raw diet as a method of food therapy with its little coeliac patients, and the medical director at that time published in a monograph an account of the "staggering success" of the cure thus

*Coeliac.—Tʀ.

achieved. As a consequence, other children's hospitals abroad have likewise tested this raw food treatment of coeliac disease and experienced the same success.

10. CURE OF FACIAL ACNE (FROM A LADY'S LETTER)

"For many years I suffered from an ugly, if harmless, facial eczema. The best doctors—and I tried so many of them—diagnosed acne, and recommended to me this and that, but I never got any help from them. During my whole youth I had to go about with this frightful facial appearance. Believe me, doctor, I would willingly have put an end to my existence, had not the thought of my mother and brothers and sisters restrained me.

"Last year (1934) came my salvation. From my married sister I got to know of your raw food diet. I quickly changed my whole method of living, and the marvel happened. My skin became quite smooth, the pimples and boils disappeared, and by the winter I was the happiest being under the sun."

Thus we see that the sole radical means of curing this skin disease, so hard for a young woman to bear, was not recommended to her by all those "so many" doctors. She came upon it accidentally, adopted it, and got well. Had she been properly fed as a child, this "disgraceful" disease, which is in point of fact a necessary regulative measure of a wrongly nourished body, would never have occurred.

Once more I ask the reader's attention to the following. Exclusively raw food diet should be employed only as a means of therapy over a limited space of time. The preservation of health is best served by a mixture of raw and cooked foods, as I have all along consistently maintained. I would ask my meat-and-wine-loving medical opponents especially to notice this point, since they are always trying to shelve the whole matter by asserting that I wish to popularize an exclusively raw diet throughout the nation. They really know perfectly well what I do want:

(i) I want the millions of invalids who have become ill through wrong feeding to be no longer treated solely by medicines and preparations, as they can recover only by means of food therapy; and

(ii) I want the prevention of many serious diseases arising from wrong feeding, which rage today and number their victims by millions, by means of a scientifically established and urgently necessary change in the people's diet, especially children's diet.

Conclusion

THE transformation in children's diet which the new era of nutritional research and my suggestions here set out wish to accomplish is something quite fundamental. It will meet with much resistance and many obstacles. Hardly anyone, I suppose, is in a better position to appreciate that fact than myself, since for forty years I have been struggling to get my teaching accepted. Yet it is a case of one thing or the other.

"Ignorance," says a great thinker among the physicians of our age, Martin Sihle, "is the cause of all disease." Truly, forty years ago we did not take into account three central problems of nutrition. We did not know what effect diet produces in the human body. We did not know the relation between food and health, or food and disease. And therefore we did not know either, that the general constitutional deterioration of civilized humanity, and a whole host of diseases, sufferings and sickness, are caused to a large extent by the diet that is thought right and proper for civilized nations, as it has developed during the epoch of progress and industrialization. We were at that time simply not in a position to recognize and to estimate the effect of this diet.

But today we are in a position to recognize all this. And it is therefore our duty as doctors not to shrink from opposition, but with all our powers to spread enlightenment, and to prepare the way for the changes that must come. Wrong feeding has its most harmful effects during the years of growth, and it is therefore here that the change is most necessary. Nothing is more important for the future of our people than that the children should be given proper, natural food. If I have won the co-operation of any of my readers in carrying out this task, I am well rewarded. To conclude with the telling words of McCarrison: "There is indeed no more important problem before the country at the present moment than the provision for the people of a properly constituted diet and no more urgent necessity than their instruction in these matters."